Why Do Men Fall Asleep After Sex?

MARK LEYNER is the author of five books: *Et Tu, Babe*; *My Cousin, My Gastroenterologist*; *Tooth Imprints on a Corn Dog*; *I Smell Esther Williams*; and *The Tetherballs of Bougainville*. He has written scripts for a variety of films and television shows. His fiction and nonfiction continues to appear regularly in *The New Yorker*, *Time*, *GQ*, and *Travel & Leisure*.

WILLIAM GOLDBERG, M.D., is a practicing physician at Bellevue Hospital and NYU Medical Center, a painter, and a writer. His paintings have been exhibited in New York City and are held in private collections in Madrid, Sydney, New York, and San Francisco.

Why Do Men Fall Asleep After Sex?

Things You'd Only Ask a Doctor After Your Third Gin 'n' Tonic

Mark Leyner and
Billy Goldberg, M.D.

An Orion paperback

First published in Great Britain in 2006
by Orion Books Ltd,
Orion House, 5 Upper St Martin's Lane,
London WC2H 9EA

1 3 5 7 9 10 8 6 4 2

A CIP catalogue record for this book is available
from the British Library.

ISBN-13 978 0 7528 8218 5
ISBN-10 0 7528 8218 X

Typeset by Geoff Green Book Design
Printed and bound in Great Britain by
Clays Ltd, St Ives plc

www.orionbooks.co.uk

This book is dedicated to all the little things that made the production of this book possible and daily life more enjoyable:

A   Ambien, Apple Computer, *American Idol*, Artichokes, Almodóvar

B   Bar Pitti, Beer, Balneol, Breakfast Burritos

C   Chocolate-covered Espresso Beans, Chewy Tiny Sweet Tarts, Cap'n Crunch, Chicken Livers

D   Diet Mountain Dew, Daytime Movies, Daydreaming

E   Egg whites, Espresso

F   Flip-Flops, French Fries, Formula One, R.W. Fassbinder, John Ford

G   Google, *Grand Theft Auto*

H   Hot Dogs from Gray's Papaya, Hot Tamales, Hou Hsiao-hsien

I   Internet, iPod, Allen Iverson

J   Joe's Pizza, Jamon y Queso, Jaromir Jagr

K   Knicks, Sandy Koufax

L   Listerine, *Law & Order (Criminal Intent)*

M   Mets, Mary's Fish Camp, Maalox, Maker's Mark, Manny Being Manny

N   *New York Times*, NPR, Nyquil, Novocaine

O   Osso Bucco, Oysters

P   Propel, Percocet, Pedro, Albert Pujols, *Project Runway*

Q   "Quail Hunting"

R   Red Wine, Red Vines, Red Bull

S   Sour Skittles, Scrabble, *Survivor*, Steak Frites, Sushi

T   Target, Tequila, Tums

U   UV Radiation, Underdog

V   Vasoline, Valvoline, Velvet Underground, Vitamin C

W   WD 40, White Castle

X   X-rated anything

Y   Yoo Hoo

Z   Zeppelin, Zzzzzzzzzzs on the couch with the baseball game burbling in the background...

Contents

Contents

Chapter 4 No, I'm Not a Veterinarian!

Contents

Chapter 5 Insemination, Gestation, and Lactation (the Preggers Chapter)

Contents

Chapter 6 Eyes, Ears, Mouth, and Nose

Chapter 7 Women Want to Know

Chapter 8 A Funny Thing Happened on the Way to the Spa

Contents

Chapter 9 Growing Pains: FAQs About Puberty and Kids

Chapter 10 Natural and Unnatural Cures That We Want You to Know About

Chapter 11 The Lost and Found Department: A Random Assortment of Questions

Contents

Chapter 12 'Tis the Season (to Ask Questions)

Acknowledgments

Billy:

To Brody Alexander Goldberg: In utero, you inspired this book, and in the flesh you continue to amaze me and your mom. I would also like to thank my parents for all their unwavering support. To David, Patty, Mara, Lily, Dana, David, Lewis and Benjamin: This ride wouldn't be as much fun without you. To Horatia: New York misses you and I miss you. To all my friends and to everyone in the Emergency Department: Thanks for the support and for keeping the abuse to a minimum.

Mark:

To my brilliant and beautiful daughter, Gaby. Miss Higley Higgs. I LOVE YOU. (I know . . . my b's 2 b.)

Together we would like to thank . . .

Amanda Urban (you're the best), Carrie Thornton, Penny Simon, Steve Ross, Jenny Frost, Jim Walsh, Jennifer Smith, Alison Schwartz, Karolina Sutton at ICM and Juliet Ewers at Orion.

Obligatory Prelude to the Foreword to the Prologue to the Preface of the Introduction

Or Does Anyone Read This Crap?

Okay, so here we go again . . .

It feels a bit different this time. When we were writing *Why Do Men Have Nipples?*, we had no idea that anyone (other than our editor, wives, moms, and dads) would read the book. Shows what we know.

Our little *Nipples* book has sold more than a million copies internationally and spent twenty-five weeks (and counting) on the *New York Times* bestseller list. You have no idea how much we have loved this ride and how much we adore babbling on TV, drive-time radio, and especially in the makeup rooms where we shamelessly flirted with a succession of fantastic makeup artists at all the major networks. (By the way, Mark prefers the spray-on nozzle method, which he likens to being wax-polished in a car wash.)

But a funny thing happened along the way. We quickly became aware of the fact that we'd barely scratched the surface. As we talked to people who'd enjoyed our first book, we began accumulating hundreds of new questions—some funny, down-to-earth, exotic, some embarrassing, some perplexing, but always thought-provoking enough that we knew we'd have to include them in a brand-new volume.

We realized the gravity of the somber task ahead of us. We felt deputized. We knew we were now bound by honor and a fiduciary duty to you, our readers, to deliver unbiased, unadulterated, thoroughly researched, and unimpeachably factual answers to your questions. Humbled, but galvanized and inspired by the immense challenge that lay before us, we hunkered down in a windowless, antiseptic research cocoon, and made a solemn pledge to produce a new volume that would surpass the original and blaze new trails in the democratization of medical knowledge . . .

Oh, please ... SEQUEL!!!!!!! Here it is ... *Why Do Men Fall Asleep After Sex?*

Leyner: You there, Nip Bro?

Gberg: Yeah.

Leyner: Just hit the motherload of medical anomalies and bizarre conditions!

Gberg: Halleluyah.

Gberg: Get us some words too!

Leyner: It's the table of contents of some obscure academic book ... but it lists everything ... we just have to pick and choose and look some shit up online ... but it's a complete list. You'll be delighted.

Gberg: You are prolific!!

Leyner: Don't worry. Soon we'll devote ourselves fully to the book. We'll get it all done ... no problem ... and have a blast too! I promise you.

Gberg: Will you promise me a rose garden?

Leyner: Alice in Wonderland syndrome!!

Leyner: People who see things in the wrong proportions ... very small or very big!!! It's an actual syndrome!!

Gberg: It wouldn't be bad to have someone with that syndrome check you out with your pants down.

Leyner: Here's a whole list of prefixes (e.g. brachi) and suffixes (e.g. plasy, algia, etc.) ... we could make a little game of create your own pathology.

Gberg: I also heard that they are changing the name of the disease Reiter's syndrome because they found out Reiter was a Nazi.

Gberg: Excellent.

Leyner: That's fantastic!!

Leyner: We should also tell some stories ...

Gberg: We only have eight weeks to finish the book.

Gberg: Tight. Very tight.

Leyner: I know. We'll do it.

Leyner: We could do the book in a month.

Gberg: It will require a lot of chocolate-covered espresso beans and diet soda.

Leyner: And we have two.

Leyner: We should really consider a research person.

Leyner: Let's talk about it on Friday ...

Gberg: Or a geisha.

Gberg: A research geisha.

Leyner: Someone to squeegee our ball sweat.

Gberg: Mine are as dry as the Gobi.

Leyner: Maybe we should even save this.

Gberg: Consider it saved.

Leyner: From now on we should save EVERY one of our IMs.

Leyner: Seriously.

Leyner: OK.

Gberg: Done!

Gberg: OK, let's talk later ...

Leyner: Later.

Leyner: Victory or Death.

Chapter 1

Battle of the Sexes

It's 9 A.M. Leyner and I are sitting in our office, awaiting our first patients.

After finishing *Why Do Men Have Nipples?*, we decided to go into practice together. Leyner's BA in English and Masters in creative writing hardly qualified him to treat patients, and his adamant refusal to seek higher medical education didn't help matters. (Leyner was violently opposed to the idea of attending school again. During a rather heated discussion on the issue, he smashed a printer we'd just purchased for our new office, and scrawled an adolescent vulgarity on a print of van Gogh's *Sunflowers* hanging in the hallway.)

When Leyner regained his composure, we realized that the thing that made our partnership work was our fanatical mutual admiration, our boundless love of arcane medical matters and our capacity to talk endlessly about our own insecurities and desires, and the personal crises and dilemmas in which life occasionally ensnares us. For some bizarre reason, people other than the two of us seem to be interested in what we have to say … We finally agreed that if Dr. Phil could do it on TV, why couldn't we offer our learned and empathic counseling services? This would preclude the need for advanced degrees, and I also figured it was a way to safely keep medical instruments and sharp surgical devices out of Leyner's emotionally unstable grasp.

Our office assistant, Wendy Thurston, who was recently fired from her position as senior editor at Half a Dozen Ponds Press after she was arrested for shoplifting lipstick from the local pharmacy, escorted our first patients of the day into our office. They were a young couple. The woman was attractive, conservatively dressed, and—at first glance—seemed somewhat despondent. Her husband, dragging behind, seemed more interested in the defaced painting in the hallway than in being here to address "issues" with his inexplicably unfulfilled wife.

"Who wrote 'sniff my crotch' on the van Gogh out there?" he asked as he took a seat next to his wife. "I love it!!!" he guffawed, slapping his thighs.

His wife grimaced with chagrin. "You see," she said, "I married a philistine and a troglodyte."

"Insult me in English, you pretentious bitch!" the husband replied.

Leyner assumed a fighting stance—the Drunken Crane pose of the Shaolin School.

I remembered the last time that Leyner assaulted a patient and, hoping to avoid more litigation, I interceded and suggested that Leyner's pose is the typical non-communicative and defensive position that spouses take and that this impedes further discussion. A disappointed Leyner shrugged in agreement and slouched into his leather armchair.

As I turned to the fuming couple, I asked them to role-play with us. I offered to play the husband to our female patient and Leyner enthusiastically embraced the opportunity to play wife to the man.

I began, "Sometimes patients feel more open and honest with a surrogate spouse, so I want you to tell me exactly what you need from me in this marriage."

Sheepishly, the woman responded, "I need a partner, a soul mate, someone to talk to. Sometimes I just want to be heard. I don't need someone to solve all my problems, I just need someone to hold me and listen." The husband jumped at the chance to answer his wife, but I stopped him.

"I want you to respond to Leyner as if he were your wife. This will keep the two of you from becoming defensive and allow you to see each other's point of view."

Confused, the husband looked at the beaming Leyner and said, "I listen, I hold you, but it's always the things that I don't do. I feel like you don't appreciate the things that I do. I barbecue, I walk the dog, I take out the garbage, I even put down the toilet seat. What do you want me to do? Lactate?"

Leyner rose from his chair, red-faced, tears welling in his eyes, spittle flying from his mouth as he gesticulated with melodramatic hysteria.

"Bastard … You stole my youth and now you're drowning my soul in your vile bullshit. You make love to me as if I were some inflatable doll—pumping for a minute or two while you watch Sky Sports and then lose consciousness. You're torturing me … I hate you. I HATE YOU!!!"

Tears streamed down Leyner's face as he wept uncontrollably. The couple sat silently, completely and utterly confused.

So much for the role-playing. Unfortunately, there is no easy solution to the Battle of the Sexes, but here are some answers …

Why do women pee more than men?

Any man who has taken a long car trip with a woman truly believes that women need to pee more than men. As we speed down the highway and begrudgingly pull into another rest stop, we wonder whether this is the result of a genetic difference, obsessive water consumption, or a vicious plan to throw us off schedule.

If you happened to be leafing through the February 5, 2005, edition of *The Journal of Urology*, you could begin to find an answer. Doctors reviewed twenty-four-hour "urinary diaries" of both men and women and recorded fluid intake and urinary frequency. They found that women do pee more often than men but not because they drink more. In fact, men generally have higher fluid intake but don't need to go as often. When men finally feel the urge, they tend to pee in higher volumes than women. This is because men have a larger bladder capacity. That means smaller bladders in the ladies. Women are also more likely to suffer from overactive bladder syndrome, which makes them go even more. No wonder the line is always longer at the ladies' room.

Diaries and memoirs are a red-hot genre these days. There's *The Diary of Anne Frank*, Che Guevara's *Motorcycle Diaries*, *The Personal Memoirs of Ulysses S. Grant*, Karrine Steffans's *Confessions of a Video Vixen*, and, of course, James Frey's *A Million Little Pieces*. But if you're inspired by literary ambition, and decide to keep and then publish your Urine Diary, be aware that it will most probably be classified as "nonfiction." You must account accurately for each and every drop, with absolutely no embellishment or hyperbole. Remember—if you fib in your Urine Diary, it could really piss off Oprah.

Why do women have smaller feet than men?

Overall, women are smaller than men. The "why" is an evolutionary question that is too complex for us to answer here. But the ways in which men and women differ anatomically is more approachable. Male and female feet differ in size relative to stature. Men of the same height as women tend to have longer and wider feet.

When you compare a male and female foot of the same size, the woman's foot will have a higher arch, a shallower first toe, a shorter ankle length, and a smaller instep. Women also have larger calf circumferences.

Women seem to have an incredible knack for disregarding the shape of their feet and forcing them into ever smaller and pointier high heels. This callous disregard makes the foot differences between the genders even greater by ultimately changing the natural shape of female feet. In 1993, it was reported by the American Orthopedic Foot and Ankle Society that 88 percent of the women surveyed wore shoes smaller than their actual foot size. No wonder our wives are constantly patching their traumatized feet with plasters and tape.

Are men better than women at math?

Danger! Danger! Answering this question incorrectly may force us to sleep on the couch with our wives beating us with the infamous Teen Talk Barbie that was programmed to say, "Math is hard!"

Harvard University president Lawrence Summers stepped into this minefield in 2005, when he suggested that biological differences might be one of the reasons that fewer women are in the fields of science and engineering. His speech led many professors to protest his statement, and others threatened to withhold donations. Several days later, Summers was forced to apologize. And he has since resigned.

So here are some facts (though these are often debated) …

The brains of men and women are definitely different. Women's brains are generally about 10 percent smaller than men's, but this is meaningless when it comes to intelligence. Men and women show no disparity in general intelligence. There are, however, some areas with slight variances. Women are better at visual memory, mathematical calculation, and get better school grades in mathematics. Men, however, are better at mentally rotating shapes, mathematical problem-solving, and score higher on mathematical word problems and on tests of mathematical reasoning.

Whether you agree or disagree on the interpretation of the available data, sociologists generally agree that social factors exaggerated any differences touted in the past. Women are clearly underrepresented in certain scientific fields such as math, engineering, and physics, but women now comprise more than 50 percent of medical students in the United States.

In the interest of gender harmony, let's create a new, politically correct, asexual Barbie who says something neutral like "Cognitively rotating abstract shapes can be a daunting task—I prefer mathematical calculation and more linguistically complex and empathy-centered forms of interpersonal communication." Fun!

Why don't men listen?

For this one, Dr. Billy exhaustively searched for an answer. How sweet would it be if there existed the perfect scientific comeback for the next time a woman screamed at you, "Why are you ignoring me!"

Well, here are the inklings of our anatomical answer ...

In the September 2005 issue of the journal *Neuroimage*, psychiatric researchers at the University of Sheffield reported that male and female voices activate distinct regions in the male brain. The scientists monitored the brain activity of twelve men as they listened to male and female voices. They found that in men, women's voices stimulate an area of the brain used for processing complex sounds, like music. Male voices, on the other hand, activate a region of the brain used for producing imagery. This may suggest that, at least for men, the female voice is more complex and more difficult to hear and understand.

But there's more ...

An earlier study in the July 2001 issue of *Radiology* also showed that men and women listen differently. In this study, researchers at Indiana University had twenty men and twenty women listening to a passage from a novel. While listening, they underwent functional magnetic resonance imaging (fMRI) of the brain. A majority of the men showed exclusive activity on the left side of the brain, but a majority of women showed activity on both sides of the brain.

Now, there is certainly more research to be done, but we can put these two pieces together and start to make a leap toward excusing occasional male lapses in listening to their female partners.

So men out there, here is our suggested comeback when you are accused of not listening: "Honey, I try so hard to listen. It's just that my brain is incapable of doing what my heart desires." (Then go back to watching football.)

Why don't women have Adam's apples?

The Adam's apple is simply a bulge in the human larynx that is made of cartilage. This area is called the thyroid cartilage because it is located right on top of the thyroid gland. If you want to get technical, you can also call it the prominentia laryngea, but Adam's apple is much more quaint, don't you think? It also is not exclusively a guy thing. Both men and women have thyroid cartilage and therefore an Adam's apple. They are about the same size until puberty, when increased testosterone causes it to grow more prominent in men.

For some women, the Adam's apple may be larger than desired. But fear not, modern plastic surgery can fix almost anything. All you need is a tracheal shave to reduce the size of the Adam's apple. This sounds like it can be done down at the corner barbershop, but it actually involves making a small incision in the throat and cutting away some of the prominent cartilage. This is one of the most common plastic surgeries for male-to-female transsexuals, unsurprisingly.

So where does the name Adam's apple come from? Most people say that it is from the notion that this bump was caused by the forbidden fruit getting stuck in the throat of Adam in the Garden of Eden. There is a problem with this theory because some Hebrew scholars believe that the forbidden fruit was the pomegranate. The Koran claims that the forbidden fruit was a banana. So take your pick—Adam's apple, Adam's pomegranate, Adam's banana. Eve clearly chewed before swallowing.

12:35 p.m.

Gberg: Hey, what was that title that the Aussie radio guy suggested?

Leyner: *You Put WHAT, WHERE?!*

Gberg: I think we should use that.

Gberg: Rectal foreign bodies are the new iPods.

Leyner: You make me laugh ...

Gberg: WE NEED TO HIRE A TEAM OF OOOMPA LOOMPAS TO HELP US RESEARCH.

12:40 p.m.

Leyner: That's what I tried to tell you a long time ago, motherfucker. Why don't we?

Leyner: Can't we find some "young person" to do the raw research and then we'll parse it and pickle it?

Gberg: Raw research?

Gberg: Sounds like a porn film.

Gberg: Subtle.

Leyner: Subtitle.

Gberg: *Raw Research*—A Nipple Brothers Production starring Lance Boyle.

Leyner: *Raw Research* ... starring the Nipple Brothers. I like that.

Gberg: Maybe we should have a Bravo show where we pick a new Nipple Brother.

Leyner: The supernumerary nipple.

Gberg: You need a catchphrase.

12:45 p.m.

Leyner: It should take place in some fetid garage meth lab in Nipple Ridge ...

Gberg: Mammary Ridge.

Leyner: Sorry ... I knew something was wrong with my geography ...

Gberg: We can make it a combo of *Project Runway* and *Biggest Loser*.

Leyner: And we get gorgeous, desperately horny actresses and models to play crystal-meth-addicted skanky girls from the Ozarks ... and ... and ... and ... they fluff us all day long ... as we decide who's gonna be the 3rd Nip Bro.

Gberg: There aren't enough good crystal-meth-addicted skanky-girl parts for actors these days.

Gberg: That should be its own category at the Oscars.

Leyner: And the winner for ... crystal-meth-addicted skanky girl ... Ooooh, I'm so nervous I can't even get my trembling, tweaking fingers to open this fucking envelope ...

12:50 p.m.

Gberg: This IM thing is dangerous. I am supposed to be researching the new temporal artery thermometer and instead I am rambling on with you.

Leyner: It's ... LISA KUDROW!!!!!!!!!!!! Mazel tov, you drooling skanky girl!!

Gberg: You need some anger management.

Leyner: YEAH, BABY!!!!

Leyner: I'll call you later.

Gberg: Ciao.

Leyner: Ciao.

Can men lactate?

You can't write a book called *Why Do Men Have Nipples?* without getting a question about lactating men. This one came during a radio interview when an irate caller insisted that a man could nurse his own child. We argued with him, but there was no convincing this guy (Benson—are you reading this?) that it was not possible.

Here is the truth. The mammary glands of human males *can* produce milk but certainly not enough to feed a child. Usually, male milk production is from a pathological condition. The most common cause of man milk is a prolactin-secreting tumor (prolactinoma) in the pituitary gland. Prolactin is a hormone that stimulates milk production. Overproduction of prolactin may be caused by some drugs, including phenothiazines, certain drugs given for high blood pressure (especially methyldopa), opioids, and even licorice. Male lactation is also caused by the hormonal treatments used in men who are suffering from prostate cancer. Doctors use female hormones to decrease the growth of the prostate, but these can also cause milk production or galactorrhea.

Extreme starvation—by radically disrupting the equilibrium of hormone production—can also make men lactate. (This has been observed in prisoners of war.)

It is also possible for males to induce lactation through constant massage and stimulation of the nipple over a long period of time, but that sounds like a lot of work.

Then there is the fruit bat. Only one male mammal, the Dayak fruit bat, is known to produce milk.

So if you are a male fruit bat with prostate cancer who likes to massage his own nipples, and you happen to be a prisoner of war, let the nursing begin.

Why do men snore more than women?

In our last book, we dispelled the myth that men fart more than women. So what about snoring? In this case, the men are guilty as charged. We do snore more for several reasons. To begin with, women have anatomically different airways than men. Women have a wider airway circumference so if there is any obstruction, there's a chance the air passing through will not be as likely to hit the oropharyngeal structures as it would in a man. Additionally, a woman's airway is less prone to collapse than a man's airway, and that works in her favor as far as snoring is concerned.

When men put on weight, they tend to put it on around the neck area, whereas women put on weight around the hips. The fatty tissue around the neck literally squeezes the airway closed so air can't pass through smoothly. Air then hits the structures within the throat and vibrates them, which causes the noise we know as snoring.

Smoking and drinking also lead to increased snoring. In general, women tend not to smoke and drink as much as men, and therefore don't suffer the snoring consequences.

Pregnant women do tend to snore more because the blood flow around the nasal area can increase, which causes the lining of the nose and throat to swell. This makes breathing more difficult, so there would be a tendency to sleep with the mouth open, giving rise to snoring.

Why do men fall asleep after sex?

Leave it to a ninety-two-year-old woman to break down a complicated question into the simplest terms. When we told Billy's wife's grandmother the name of our new book, she answered in a second, "Because they work so damn hard!"

As much as we would have liked to settle on that answer, we knew more was needed to make our editor happy. So we scoured the medical literature to try to put this issue to rest. We found studies with fornicating rats, hamsters, and prairie voles, but there was very little direct information about the postcoital snooze. There are many hormonal changes that occur with orgasm and some of these changes may offer an explanation for why men fall asleep.

After orgasm, both men and women release the chemicals oxytocin, prolactin, gamma amino butyric acid (GABA), and endorphins. Each of these contributes to that roll-over-and-snore feeling. They seem to be secreted in equal amounts in men and women, but we all know who orgasms more frequently.

The hormone oxytocin is known to have several effects, including establishment of maternal behavior, stimulation of uterine smooth muscle contraction at birth, and stimulation of milk ejection (milk letdown). It is also referred to as the "cuddling hormone" since it tends to elicit the need to be close and bond but not in a sexual way. In one study, oxytocin was shown to inhibit male sexual behavior in prairie voles. Maybe it's the oxytocin that makes us feel satiated and rested after a good romp.

Prolactin is another player in the sex/sleep conundrum. It is produced in the pituitary gland and its best known function is the stimulation of milk production. Prolactin is believed to relieve sexual arousal after orgasm and take your mind off sex. Levels of prolactin rise during sleep, and some patients with prolactin-secreting tumors report frequent sleepiness. So prolactin seems like it may be a culprit too.

Gamma amino butyric acid (GABA) and endorphins also have a calming effect and may make you pass out post-sex.

The tantric answer is that the male orgasm releases outward energy or jing, while the female orgasm is an inward explosion.

Last but not least, we have Grandma's reasoning. It is thought that exertion during sex and after climax depletes the muscles of energy-producing glycogen. This leaves men feeling sleepy. Since men have more muscle mass than women, men become more tired after sex. Also (believe it or not!) women don't always have an orgasm, and that keeps them from producing all those other hormones we just talked about.

Hmmm ... maybe Grandma was right.

9:53 a.m.

Gberg: Good morning.

Leyner: Good morning ... won't you light my candle????

Gberg: We need to figure out the new title.

Gberg: You didn't like *Why Do Women Have Voiding Dysfunction and De Novo Detrusor Instability After Colposuspension?*

Leyner: I e-mailed you asking how you could have kept that pithy, memorable, ultra-catchy piece of pop heroin to yourself all this time.

Leyner: Did you see any of the whole Oprah drama/debacle?

9:55 a.m.

Gberg: Yeah, who cares if Frey duped his readers. Are you worried that we are next? Afraid she is going to confront us on the veracity of our books?

Leyner: I can't wait to be confronted on the veracity of anything and everything I've ever written. That guy is such a pathetic abject pussy ...

Gberg: James Frey? Yeah, but he is a very rich pussy now!

Leyner: I've NEVER told the truth in my life. EVER. It's my badge of honor. As a thief and a renegade.

Gberg: I can hear "Born to Be Wild" playing in the background.

Gberg: That or some Debbie Gibson song.

Leyner: Someone was complaining that even after (or because) of that telehumiliation, he's numero uno on Amazon this morning ... And this indignant commentator went on to say ...

Leyner: We live in a time when even the endorsement of Osama bin Laden can make a book a bestseller!

Leyner: I want some Chechen mafioso to endorse our new book.

Gberg: It doesn't matter what they say. If the book is mentioned on TV, there is a Pavlovian response to buy.

Gberg: We need endorsements from labor unions and gay rights groups.

Leyner: Did you read about that new prion disease in deer ... Some sort of "wasting" disease ... but they think its etiology is similar to mad cow ...

10:00 a.m.

Gberg: Sounds like the beginning of a bad science joke.

Leyner: We need endorsement from Hamas.

Leyner: If you can't go out with your crossbow and impale Bambi's dad and then go home and butcher and gorge on it with a bunch of inbred

Appalachian hydrocepahlic morons and NOT
have the expectation of safety and healthy
good eatin' ... then this country is going to
fucking hell in a handbasket, my friend.

Gberg: That sounds like an ad campaign for
Appalachian travel.

Leyner: Hey ... if we mention Appalachian travel
in the new book ... maybe we'll all get free travel and accommodations to ... APPALACHIA!!!!!
You, me, and the girls!!!!!!!

Gberg: Yeah, baby.

Gberg: Back to the title. I am not a big fan of the
new one.

Leyner: We can hunt and drink ... kinda
Brokeback, dude ... catchin' the vibe?

Gberg: Back off.

Leyner: Just testing the waters ...

10:05 a.m.

Leyner: *Why Do Men Pass Out After Sex?*

Leyner: I could live with it. But ... tell me what
other people said about it.

Gberg: I researched the sleep and sex thing and
there isn't any good answer. We can talk about
different hormones and tantric sex but no
clear science.

Leyner: Let's look into it a little more before we
toss it ... there's something appealing about it
to me ... and this is after I was VERY skeptical
about it ... but it sort of "grew on me."

Gberg: Like a fungus.

Gberg: Hey, give me a call at home, let's talk, and then I have to go to work.

Leyner: We don't talk enough about fungal infections.

Leyner: I mean our society as a whole.

Gberg: Onychomycosis.

10:10 a.m.

Gberg: Mycotic aneurysms.

Leyner: Es-plain that to me. What sort of infection is that?

Gberg: *My Cousin Vinny.*

Leyner: Ooooh, Doctor ... talk dirty to me ...

Gberg: Onychomycosis=nail fungus.

Leyner: Oh ... right ... nail fungus!!

Leyner: Good!

Gberg: Beware the manicure/pedicure with dirty tools.

Leyner: Is this in the book?

Gberg: There is one question about pedicures, I think.

Gberg: I will check.

Gberg: Give me a call so I can start my day.

Leyner: You're not implying that all those cute adorable luscious, lusting Korean manicurists are in this country at the behest of the evil Kim Jong-il in order to spread onychomycosis to all Americans, are you?

Gberg: Exactly.

Leyner: OK, I'll call you in a moment or two. Bye-bye, birdie.

Gberg: Adios.

Gberg: Wish I could say goodbye in Korean.

Leyner: Wait, I was just reading Carrie's e-mail.

Gberg: And?

Leyner: I'm going to write her back that I much prefer "pass out."

Gberg: I think fall asleep is fine. I prefer it to pass out.

Leyner: I know you do. Tell her. Let her sort it all out.

Gberg: She is interested in seeing the intros we wrote. Should we send them, or should we make her suffer and wait to the last minute to see everything?

Gberg: I know how you like to torture her.

Leyner: I don't have a problem with her reading what we wrote the other day. Let's send them. You agree?

Gberg: Yes. What was that thing you read in the paper that you wanted me to look at?

Leyner: It was in yesterday's *New York Times* ...

Leyner: "Scientists Find Gene That Controls Type of Earwax in People."

Gberg: You should have been an earwax geneticist!

Leyner: I also want to add a castration/voice-change question.

Gberg: We should have a whole eunuch chapter.

Leyner: Earwax geneticist? It's never too late ... but I don't want to go back to school, remember?

Gberg: Maybe even write a whole eunuch book and a sitcom.

Gberg: You can get any degree online.

Leyner: Maybe we should have a patient see us who just wants them cut off ... y'know can't deal with the desire and futile search for a mate, etc., etc.

Gberg: Don't joke. Remember the story of the schizophrenic guy who cut his off.

Leyner: Self-orchi-something or other ...

Gberg: No, a guy who I saw at the hospital who cut off his penis and flushed it down the toilet.

Leyner: What's the fancy-shmancy word for removal of the testicle ...? It's orch-something.

Gberg: Orchiectomy.

Gberg: Sounds like a pasta.

Leyner: Thanks, Chief.

Gberg: Chef.

Do men sleep more than women?

Are those men who conked out after sex *still* asleep?

Actually, some authorities believe that women are biologically programmed to sleep better than men. Estrogen tends to decrease the number of awakenings after you finally fall asleep and also increases total sleep time. Unfortunately, menopause and pregnancy throw off this advantage.

In the Bruskin Research survey of 1,000 Americans aged eighteen and older, one in five men aged eighteen to thirty-four conceded they take longer than an hour to fall asleep. Also, more than 30 percent of men in that age group admitted to falling asleep at work, clearly making up for time lost during their primary nocturnal sleep.

As we discussed earlier, snoring and sleep-disordered breathing is more common in men than women and this also adds to the dozing dysfunction of men.

Researching this one's made me a little sleepy. I think it's time for a nap …

Do men have shorter attention spans than women?

We've been trying to answer this question for weeks now, but we can't seem to concentrate long enough to write anything.

One thing that we do know for certain is that attention-deficit hyperactivity disorder (ADHD) occurs primarily in males. The male-to-female ratio has been reported to be as high as nine to one.

Did you ever notice that … squirrels never fall out of trees … and where do all the dead pigeons go? … Uh … wait … weren't we supposed to be answering a question about … what was it … ?

Actually, there's no more information about gender differences in attention spans, so you'll have to ponder this one on your own.

Why do women live longer than men?

Life expectancy varies from country to country and people definitely live longer in developed nations than in the Third World. But one of the constants in almost all countries is that women outlive men. In the United States, the average life expectancy for men is 74.5 years, while women can expect to be around for 79.9 years.

There are many theories about the reason for female longevity, and since a complete answer would require an entire book, we will try to summarize. There really are two separate questions:

1. Why do men die so young?
2. Why do women live so long?

The available evidence points toward evolution, behavior, and biology. In terms of evolution, women are helped by the need to live long enough to raise their children, while men wear themselves out competing for the right to procreate. Behavioralists point out that around the time of puberty through the twenties, men are three times more likely to die than women. Most of the male fatalities are caused by reckless behavior or violence. In the older age group, behavior-related fatalities are still more common among men. Illnesses related to smoking and alcohol consumption also kill more men than women. Lastly, there are some strong biological factors that favor women. Heart disease targets men more readily, and is the main cause of the gender gap in this arena.

The gender discrepancy is most pronounced in the very old. Among centenarians worldwide, women outnumber men nine to one. The good news for the men out there is that if you make it past a hundred, you will definitely have your pick of the litter at the nursing home.

• Chapter 2 •

In the Kitchen

I t's another day at the office and Leyner has yet to
arrive. Our first appointment is with Judd Wilson.
(Names are changed to comply with patient-privacy
regulations.) Judd suffers from body dysmorphic disorder, a condition in which the patient has an overwhelming preoccupation with a slight or completely imagined
defect in his appearance. We've been seeing him for
several months. Although he is a fairly slender man
with a fit-looking physique, Judd is convinced that he
is not only overweight, but morbidly obese. He has
consequently developed severe eating problems, frequently starving himself and then binging uncontrollably. He was depressed and socially thwarted by his
condition. But we are making significant, albeit slow
progress. Leyner has actually developed a special relationship with Judd as he identifies with his obsessive

mirror-gazing. Right now, I need to cover for Leyner's absence.

"He's attending the annual meeting on cognitive-behavioral body-image therapy for body dysmorphic disorder in Kuala Lumpur," I say. "He definitely would be here if he could. So how have you managed this week?"

Judd tenses with frustration. "I can't take it. Food is everywhere. I am haunted by Subway sandwiches, and Mary Kate and Ashley Olsen. Just when I finally can find a balance between starving myself and overeating, I hear commercials screeching about chicken livers and Cracker Jacks."

"Well, Judd, you need to find places of safety. Places where you can escape the pressures and find your own equilibrium." I continue, "So let's try something. Start with this office. Let's make it your refuge. In here, there is no pressure. No commercials. No posters. Nothing to resist, nothing to indulge."

Somewhat more relaxed, Judd responds, "That feels good. I like that."

At that very moment, Leyner bursts through the door clutching a large greasy brown sack. "Dude, sorry I'm late," he says, as he voraciously tears into an overflowing bucket of fried chicken.

Suddenly, he stops eating and looks up at me, and then Judd, his brow knit with consternation.

"This is wrong … I'm sorry … How could I? … What was I thinking?" he stammers.

"It's okay," replies an ashen-faced Judd.

"No, how could I …? How could I eat fried chicken without …"

He reaches into the sack and triumphantly pulls out a large oily container.

"… without curly fries!!!!"

Now totally pale, Judd shrieks, "But this is my safe place!"

Leyner, without missing a beat, flings a half-eaten drumstick at Judd and snarls, "Buddy, how many times have I told you, the world is a gauntlet, a lifelong, sadistic, hazing ritual, a minefield fraught with agonizing death at every turn." Saying this, Leyner begins shoveling heaped spoonfuls of tapioca pudding into his mouth.

Judd, now beside himself with rage, begins to get up from the sofa.

Seeing an opening, I intercede. "Judd, do you see our method? Can it be any more clear? The point we're trying to dramatize here is that you can never effectively protect yourself from your own innate desires and feelings. You need to confront, honor, and sometimes actually indulge your fears. Like the anger you're feeling right now. Throw that drumstick back at Leyner. And tell me how it feels."

He picks up the gnawed chicken leg and hurls it violently at Leyner's head. Like a Frisbee-catching Jack Russell terrier, Leyner adroitly catches the drumstick in his teeth and begins to laugh hysterically, as tapioca spurts from his nostrils.

"Man, *that* is refreshing, I can breathe again. Thanks, Doc."

Leyner strides from the office, inhaling and exhaling with great gusto and satisfaction.

I watch his triumphant exit and turn to see Judd laughing along. Somehow Leyner's unorthodox methodology has succeeded, and the now ebullient Judd just wants to know one thing: Why *does* food come out of your nose when you laugh while eating? This, I can answer.

Is it true that an apple a day keeps the doctor away?

It certainly would be great to spend your money on apples rather than health insurance. Unfortunately, an apple a day will not keep you totally disease-free, but there is some evidence that it can help.

Scientists have done many studies looking for a specific chemical in apples that could prove this old adage. Quercetin, a polyphenolic compound (polyphenols are the antioxidant compounds found in red wine), is the compound most referenced for its curative properties. Quercetin was found to help in lung and prostate cancer and to reduce the incidence of cardiovascular disease. Apples also contain other antioxidant compounds and fiber. The peel has the highest proportion of these antioxidants (almost five times greater), so definitely don't skip the peel. There has also been some research that has found that apples help in fighting Alzheimer's and breast cancer.

Researchers in Canada looked at eight varieties of apple and found that Red Delicious and Northern Spy apples had the highest levels of antioxidant chemicals. This study left out many varieties that are also popular, so your favorite may still be good for you.

It is no magic bullet, but hey, it makes apple pie sound more nutritious, right?

Does milk cause an increase in mucus?

This is definitely going to be one of those questions that will cause us some trouble. People insist that milk causes increased mucus and most don't like it when their entrenched beliefs are contradicted by science.

Milk does not cause increased mucus production. Several studies confirm the fact that milk is not the bad guy many "lactophobes" make it out to be. What these phlegmy people are probably feeling is milk coating the throat, causing the sensation of increased phlegm. When milk was compared with liquids of similar viscosity, there was no difference in mucus quantities. Whatever symptoms people feel should go away shortly after the coating dissipates.

So, if you're still feeling phlegmy or hawking up spit, don't blame it on the poor hardworking dairy cows. They are just doing their job.

Is the red dye in maraschino cherries really bad for you?

Or do you suffer from erythrophobia?

Erythrophobia refers to an abnormal and persistent fear of blushing, but also refers to a fear of the color red. It is not surprising that someone could associate the color red with fear. There certainly are a great many scary "reds"—the Red Scare of the 1950s, Communism, of course, redcoats, getting caught red-handed, being in the red, taking the red-eye, a code red, and red flags are just a few.

No wonder people think that red maraschino cherries are dangerous.

Food colorants have been used for many years. Some historians believe that they were first used around 1500 bc. In 1938, the Federal Food, Drug, and Cosmetic Act was passed, giving the FDA the authority to oversee the safety of food, drugs, and cosmetics. This is the origin of "FD&C" that you see before a dye's number on product labels in the USA. In 1960, an amendment was added to the Food, Drug, and Cosmetic Act. This was called the Delaney Clause and it prohibited the marketing of any color additive that was found to cause cancer in animals or humans, regardless of amount. Since then, Red #1, #2, and #4 have all been banned in America. The two main red dyes that are still used are Red #3 and Red #40. Both are used in maraschino cherries.

Are these dyes perfectly safe? The cancer risks for Red #3 are as small as one in a hundred thousand over a seventy-year period. These dyes are found in many foods so an occasional maraschino cherry probably isn't going to increase your risk. But if you're scarfing down several whole jars a day, you might want to consider switching to olives.

Will a watermelon bush grow in your belly if you swallow a watermelon seed?

We have been asked several versions of this question and have resisted our desire to purge it from the book entirely, because the answer seems SO obvious. Of course you won't grow a watermelon bush, a cherry tree, or a pumpkin patch in your stomach if you swallow seeds.

Even if you clamp your duodenum, eat a bag of potting soil, swallow seeds, and then top it off with a shot or two of Miracle-Gro, nothing will grow. The stomach is hardly fertile ground for agriculture.

Why do you lose your sense of taste when your nose is stuffed?

Humans are microsmatic, which means that we have poorly developed olfactory organs. For us, the sense of smell is not essential for survival as it is for other animals, and smell always seems to take a back seat to the other senses. Sight and hearing have always appeared to be the most necessary senses for humans, and touch and taste are often thought to be more significant than smell. But what is taste without smell? Pretty limited, actually.

Humans can recognize as many as 10,000 different scents. Taste, on the other hand, is limited to four basic categories: sweet, salty, sour, and bitter. Around 75 percent of what we perceive as taste actually comes from our sense of smell. Food gives off odor molecules that our brain recognizes. So it is no surprise that when your nose is stuffed, your taste suffers.

Why does spinach leave a chalky taste in your mouth?

We tried to answer this question in *Why Do Men Have Nipples?*, but it was difficult to find a clear answer so we just left it on the cutting-room floor. Well, after many plates of sautéed spinach at one of our favorite restaurants, Bar Pitti in New York, we needed to find an answer.

Spinach is a famously healthy food due in great part to Popeye. (In our humble opinions, the greatest incarnations of Popeye are the original E. C. Segar cartoons that appeared in newspapers in the 1930s and the fantastic original animated versions by the Fleischer Brothers, but we digress.)

The most likely cause for the spinach aftertaste is the large amount of calcium, specifically calcium oxalate, found in spinach. You also will find the same compound in beet greens and rhubarb, so you'll encounter the same aftertaste when eating these delicious foods.

Does barbecuing cause cancer?

Picture this. A large man in plaid shorts stands beside his barbecue grill. His round beer belly is pushing out against his apron, which reads, "Will Grill for Sex." An enormous flame is rising up in the air and the meat is crackling its way to an indistinguishable black-encrusted mess. The problem is that this familiar but unpleasant sight might actually be dangerous.

Studies have found that two types of cancer-causing agents can be formed during barbecuing. These are polycyclic aromatic hydrocarbons (PAHs) and heterocyclic amines (HCAs). PAHs (mainly benzopyrene) are formed in smoke and are found on the surface of the meat and can be fairly easily scraped off.

HCAs are found inside the meat. They are caused by putting the meat under high temperatures and can also be formed in a frying pan or oven, as well as the grill.

Don't worry, there's still hope for all you backyard barbecue big shots. We can control how we cook to minimize the risk.

Here are some grilling tips:

- Marinate.
- Precook food before grilling. (This reduces the exposure to high heat, and you can drain fat to have less dripping and smoking.)
- Flip often.

- Cook at lower temperatures.
- Don't cook directly over coals.
- Limit use of the lid to reduce cooking in smoke.
- Remove any blackened parts on the surface of the meat.

Why does food come out of your nose when you laugh while eating?

The answer to this question is a simple anatomy lesson. The nose and the mouth are connected inside the back of the throat (the pharynx). The soft palate and the uvula move up, back, and out of the way when swallowing to allow food or drink to go down unimpeded. In this position, the soft palate also blocks the passage of air back out through the nose. When you are not swallowing, the soft palate and uvula go back in their regular position, allowing air to pass freely in and out through the nose into the pharynx.

So what happens when that geyser of milk comes through your nose? If you start laughing after swallowing, the uvula and palate return to their resting positions to let the air out. The pressure of laughing forces the milk out through the pharynx and into the nose and presto ... the dreaded Milk Nose!

Is coffee good for your memory?

Caffeine is the world's most widely used stimulant. It has been studied for its relationship with a remarkable number of conditions. When we searched for articles pertaining to coffee or caffeine in a medical database, there were almost twenty thousand references from the past forty years.

While many links between coffee and various cancers have been suggested, most evidence shows no connection between coffee intake and cancer of the oral cavity, esophagus, stomach, liver, breast, ovary, kidney, and pancreas. There is a possible increased risk of bladder cancer with heavy coffee intake, but a slightly decreased incidence of colon cancer. In the end, there seems no real reason to change your habits.

Now back to the question: Some studies have shown drinking coffee may help improve memory because it leads to increased attention and arousal. Investigators postulate that it can have a temporary effect on the growth of the nerve cells in the brain, specifically the spine-like structures on the nerve cells (dendrites). The effects of increased attention and arousal are only temporary and may be less significant in habitual coffee-drinkers.

Why do wintergreen Life Savers spark when you bite them?

For those of you who have never experienced this phenomenon, just turn off the lights, look into the mirror, and bite down on some wintergreen Life Savers. The result: your own oral light show.

Yes, there is actually some science behind this phenomenon. It's called triboluminescence. This is a fancy way of saying the creation of light by friction. When the sugar crystals in a mint fracture, small electrical fields are created. Basically, small molecules are crashing together and this results in the creation of ultraviolet light. The bluish color you see comes from the wintergreen flavoring (methyl salicylate).

Is it true that you shouldn't drink grapefruit juice if you are taking medication?

Grapefruit juice is one of those things that you either really love or really hate. Grapefruit has a distinctive and often bitter taste, but it really depends on what type you are eating or drinking, as red are generally sweeter than white.

Grapefruit is historically a relatively young fruit. It was first discovered around 1750 in Barbados and was originally called the "forbidden fruit." Since then, it has become ubiquitous. In the 1970s, grapefruit was quite the rage with a popular grapefruit diet and many homes boasted a variety of grapefruit knives, spoons, and bowls.

But if you are a grapefruit-hater, you may have good reason to avoid it.

Interactions between grapefruit juice and medications have been recognized since about 1989, when they were discovered accidentally during an unrelated experiment.

Now for the simplified science. The chemicals in grapefruit juice inhibit an enzyme system found in the intestine that breaks down some drugs before they are absorbed into the bloodstream. If combined with grapefruit juice, these drugs pass through untouched, allowing a higher amount to reach the bloodstream. This leads to higher levels of the drug in the blood, and higher levels may cause significant side effects. But not all drugs are broken down by the enzyme system that grapefruit juice blocks. Common drugs that are affected by grapefruit juice include the blood-thinner Coumadin, some blood-pressure-lowering pills, seizure medication, cholesterol-lowering drugs, and Viagra. If you are taking any prescription drugs, just ask your doctor or pharmacist and they can check for interactions.

Are blueberries good for your memory?

I, Billy, often tell a story about one of the nurses from the ER where I work who said that she was trying to take ginkgo biloba to improve her memory. She told me that the only problem was that she kept forgetting to take it.

Everyone is searching for the perfect memory enhancer. The list of foods that are mentioned as memory helpers is a long one, including broccoli, carrots, onions, tomatoes, apples, pomegranates, soybeans, oysters, turkey, salmon, tuna, peanuts, almonds, and, yes, blueberries.

When it comes to fruit and vegetables, blueberries have some real potential. Blueberries are one of the richest sources of antioxidants. The specific compounds they contain are called anthocyanins. If you are an aficionado of antioxidant literature, you may also know that anthocyanins are a class of polyphenolic flavonoids. (If you read *OK!* magazine, you only know that Jennifer Flavin is the wife of Sylvester Stallone.) The antioxidants in blueberries have been shown to be present in the brains of long-lived rats, and although there isn't a great deal of research on the long-term antiaging benefits, recent studies have shown blueberries protect against or reverse some age-related memory loss.

In contrast, here are some things better off forgotten:

- the time your grandma kissed you on the mouth.
- the Steven Seagal solo album (yes, the martial arts guy), *Songs from the Crystal Cave*.
- the time you fumbled hopelessly trying to unhook your first bra.
- the Federal government's response to Hurricane Katrina.

Is green tea really good for you?

This was a question that I really wanted to answer. I love a good sushi meal followed by a nice cup of green tea. What could be better than to find out that I aid my health with my own gluttony? So I searched for green tea in the medical database and hospital library and found 231 articles in the past year and a half. After leafing through reams of research, these were some of my favorite answers:

- Catechin, an ingredient of green tea, protects murine microglia from oxidative stress-induced DNA damage and cell-cycle arrest.
- Green tea extract and epigallocatechin-3-gallate, the major tea catechin, exert oxidants but lack antioxidant activities.
- Hepatoprotective effect of green tea (*Camellia sinensis*) extract against tamoxifen-induced liver injury in rats.
- Protective effect of green-tea polyphenols on the SH-SY5Y cells against 6-OHDA-induced apoptosis through ROS-NO pathway.

And:

• Paris Hilton thinks green tea is "Hot!"

Confused? The bottom line is that there are many claims that green-tea consumption can reduce cancer risk, but the evidence is not abundantly clear. There is, though, more substantive evidence that it can help lower cholesterol. So we can safely say that green tea is certainly better for you than green beer on St. Patrick's Day.

Can you drink a gallon of milk in an hour?

On call-in radio shows, we are frequently asked whether it is possible to drink a gallon of milk in an hour. Billy insists that is not part of the medical-school curriculum and that he has never treated anyone in the ER for milk-guzzling complications.

There is no doubt that drinking so much milk would be difficult, but there is no medical reason why it would be impossible. Have you ever seen those eating contests where 132-pound Japanese superstar Takeru Kobayashi eats fifty-three and a half Nathan's Famous hot dogs and buns in twelve minutes?

One warning, though … If you are a batboy, you may want to avoid attempting to drink a gallon of milk in an hour. Los Angeles Dodgers pitcher Brad Penny offered a Florida Marlins batboy $500 if he could drink a gallon of milk in under an hour without throwing up. The unidentified batboy not only failed in the attempt, but was suspended for six games.

In the *Miami Herald*, Penny summed it up perfectly: "It's kind of ridiculous that you get a ten-game suspension for steroids and a six-game suspension for milk."

• Chapter 3 •

The Wide World of Sports and Exercise

I had reservations about hiring Wendy Thurston after her shoplifting charges were dropped, but Leyner insisted that we give her a second chance. What we didn't know was that she also had a restraining order placed against her by the entire NY Rangers hockey team. We found this out when third-line center Stanislav Javenuski arrived for his sports psychology session. Leyner and I were sitting in the office reviewing our notes when we heard a ruckus and moaning emanating from the waiting room. To our surprise, when we opened the door, Wendy had Javenuski's dress-shirt yanked over his head and she was pummeling the hapless goon with punch after punch, screaming, "You wanna go? You wanna go????!!!!!!!!!" Keep in mind that the bald-headed, toothless Javenuski is considered one of the NHL's most feared enforcers. Leyner and I pulled Wendy off the bloodied Pole and escorted him into the office, while Wendy shouted, "That's right, sissy boy, into the penalty box you go!"

Javenuski had sought our guidance to overcome his overwhelming tendency to weep after a lost face-off. Hypnosis, biofeedback, and behavioral modification had all failed him and, tragically, Leyner was his last resort. I began to speak to Javenuski about other athletes who'd surmounted similar difficulties, like Chuck Knoblauch, who was unable to toss the ball to first base on routine fielding plays, Junior Totimofu, the Samoan running back, who refused to cross the seven-yard line because of the death of his pet lizard, Snowball, at the age of seven, and various other players who were unable to fulfill the most basic athletic tasks despite being paid zillions of dollars a year to do just that. Leyner interrupted and handed Javenuski a pamphlet entitled "You and Your Frontal Lobotomy."

Javenuski seemed puzzled. I shared his confusion.

Leyner stood up, grabbed Javenuski by the collar, and started buffing his forehead with a chamois that he pulled from his bag. I saw the quizzical look in our patient's eyes but tried to calm him and said, "Just be patient," as I glared at Leyner. "Go with it, pay attention to what you are feeling," I added.

"Wax on, wax off," Leyner remarked enigmatically. "Never forget the teachings of Mr. Miyagi."

At that, our toothless warrior jumped to his feet and in a strong Polish accent said, "I pay five hundred dollars for you spit-shine my head!"

An indignant Leyner brandished a letter-opener and held it menacingly to the Pole's gleaming pate. "It's all in the frontal lobes. All the emotions. I can cure your problem right here, right now, with one sharp jab of this baby right up through your sinuses. Or—as Chrissie Hynde is fond of saying—you can stop all your sobbing, and we can spend the five hundred dollars you owe us on beer and kielbasa sausage around the corner. Your call, big guy."

I gave Javenuski a sympathetic look and he shrugged.

At that, Leyner pulled another letter-opener out and slapped it in Javenuski's palm.

"Now we're going to have a face-off!"

I was prepared for the worst, but to my surprise, Javenuski started laughing hysterically, bear-hugged Leyner, and the two of them scurried off to share a sausage.

Does that black stuff athletes wear under their eyes really stop sun glare?

There's nothing like that macho ritual of American football and baseball players smearing grease under their eyes like tribal warriors preparing for battle. It just gets the competitive juices flowing.

Who knew that the stuff actually worked? Straight from the *Archives of Ophthalmology* in July 2003, Drs. Pahk and DeBroff found that the black grease used under athletes' eyes does indeed reduce glare and improve contrast sensitivity in conditions of sunlight exposure. Here's how: normally when sun shines on a person's face, the light reflects off the cheeks and straight into the eyes. The dark eye paint worn by athletes absorbs sunlight, and thus less light is reflected into the players' eyes.

Bright-red lipstick, however, has no proven benefit in improving athletic performance. So if your favorite macho athlete starts wearing that, it's okay to wonder.

Do those nose strips really work?

Have you seen these nose strips, or shall we say adhesive external nasal-dilator strips? They have been around since the late 1990s and their use has become widespread in sports. The strips stick to the outside of the nose and plastic springs in the tape spread out the nostrils. The manufacturers claim that they can give you a competitive edge by opening the nasal passages, mechanically lowering nasal airflow resistance and therefore improving performance by increasing the amount of oxygen delivered to muscle. Sounds easy.

Unfortunately, scientific studies have failed to show any significant improvement in the amount of oxygen you receive, your endurance, recovery, or overall performance.

Some studies have also been done in racehorses and here there appears to be some proof that they work better in horses. There is a debate.

These strips were originally approved for the temporary relief of breathing difficulties due to deviated nasal septum. They do seem to work for some snorers. This has been confirmed during sleep testing and measured by a respiratory-disturbance index (RDI).

So, if you are a big snorer, a racehorse, or you just don't care what the scientific evidence proves, go ahead and tape up your nose.

Does Gatorade work better to quench thirst?

We shamelessly promoted Propel Fitness Water in our last book and hope that this won't compromise the integrity of our answer here since Gatorade makes

Propel. Writing a book can be exhausting, and we hydrate with Propel, not because of any science, but because it tastes sweet like candy and we love it!

In order to get a more objective answer, we consulted one of Billy's colleagues who just completed her fellowship in sports medicine. She confirmed that there is some evidence that Gatorade and other sports drinks do offer some benefit for extra-thirsty folks.

These beverages don't necessarily hydrate better than water, but you are more likely to drink larger volumes (because they taste better than old, boring H2O), which leads to better hydration.

1:34 p.m.
Gberg: Leyner!

1:35 p.m.
Gberg: What's happenin'?
Leyner: I'm dysthymic and dysphoric and horny and HUNGRY.
Gberg: 2 Ds and 2 Hs. Good.
Leyner: You know if you're a Hell's Angel you get a merit badge for performing certain unspeakable sexual acts ...
Leyner: How come they don't award badges like that in the Boy Scouts?
Gberg: Must you be so vulgar?

Leyner: I'm going to go get some more coffee and snort another line of freeze-dried desiccated aardwolf gland ... be right back.

Gberg: I will be waiting.

Leyner: Be right back, Bunny.

Gberg: Don't "Bunny" me.

Leyner: Why? I don't mind when people call me "Misty."

Leyner: Hey ... y'ever treat someone who'd been "peppered" with bird shot?

Gberg: That is really the best story ever!

Leyner: Waiters should stroll by your table and offer freshly ground bird shot for your fettuccine.

Gberg: I can't wait to see how Jon Stewart mocks Cheney tonight.

Leyner: Imagine ... we have a vice president who shoots his own friends in the face ... HUNTING. It's like Elmer Fudd!!

Gberg: Guns don't kill people ... Big fat lying neocon scumbags kill people.

1:45 p.m.

Leyner: That's great!!! Let's make T-shirts. We'll sell them at the Nipples Brothers conventions in the future ... I sort of imagine us like William Shatner and Leonard Nimoy from *Star Trek* when we're old ... attending Nipples conventions ... People will dress as us ...

Gberg: What are you working on now?

Gberg: We really need a TV show. Not that anyone would watch, but we would have a great
time.

Leyner: What am I working on?????

Leyner: The onerous, cash-grab of a sequel ...
What do you think I'm "working" on?

Gberg: I have to keep track of your progress. The
book is due in 3 weeks. I don't want you spending another 6 hours researching anal sacs of
muskrats.

Gberg: And aardwolves.

Leyner: Did you know that even motile single-cell
organisms release pheromones to attract other
organisms?

Gberg: Did you know that temporary genital
numbness is a common side effect of long-
distance cycling?

1:50 p.m.

Gberg: Temporary Genital Numbness is a good
name for a band.

Leyner: So ... in a sense ... not to get too meta-
physical on you ... we are ALL evolved from
single-cell anal sacs!! And you talk about
INTELLIGENT DESIGN!!

Leyner: Maybe that's why Sheryl Crowe ditched
Lance.

Gberg: Ouch.

Leyner: Maybe he was too numb.

Leyner: Genital numbness is not a problem I've

experienced.

Gberg: Temporary, my friend. I am sure his perineal sensation is outstanding. I refuse to mock Lance.

Leyner: They'd have to shoot my johnson full of Lidocaine with a vet's syringe to numb that bad boy.

Gberg: Here is another great study—nocturnal penile tumescence and rigidity testing in bicycling patrol officers.

Leyner: Nor, by the way ... do I "fall asleep after sex."

Leyner: THAT's fantastic!!!!!

Leyner: Sounds like some Benny Hill skit!!!

Gberg: If it isn't embarrassing enough to be a bicycle cop.

Leyner: It's better than being a tricycle cop ... THAT's the worst!!

Gberg: This article is great. They monitored the tricycle cops during a sleep session with something called the RigiScan Plus Rigidity Assessment System.

1:55 p.m.

Leyner: Sounds like those vocational tests they used to give us in school to see if we were oriented toward any one profession.

Gberg: I can't believe some of these studies. They are almost as wild as your fiction.

Leyner: Do they hook them up to something?

Gberg: What career did they suggest for you?

Leyner: We should volunteer ... make some extra cash.

Gberg: You could be a RigiScan technician.

Leyner: I always scored very high for forensic entomologist.

Leyner: Always had a soft spot in my heart for putrescence and maggots.

Gberg: I am getting a little teary here.

Leyner: So many sexual things occur in men when they are unconscious ... it really says something about us.

Leyner: Wet dreams, nocturnal tumescence, morning erections ... it's like preying mantises ... The males keep copulating even after they're decapitated by their lovers.

2:00 p.m.

Gberg: I love the word "tumescence."

Gberg: "Senescence" also is a good one.

Leyner: I prefer the word "TURGID." It evokes the sort of erection one might get listening to Led Zeppelin ...

Gberg: I need to get a Valentine's gift for Jessica. I hate that Hallmark holiday.

Leyner: Get her Led Zep's *How the West Was Won*.

Leyner: Jimmy Page is my idol.

Gberg: Maybe she is going to get me a RigiScan Plus Rigidity Assessment System.

Leyner: (And Robespierre, of course.)

Gberg: Do you watch *American Idol*?

Leyner: That would be a sweet gift ... fer sure.

Gberg: Imagine Jimmy Page on *American Idol*.

Leyner: No ... just *Project Runway* ... that show with Clinton and what's her face where they throw people's wardrobes in the garbage ... and all *Law & Order* permutations.

2:05 p.m.

Gberg: How was your Triad DVD that you bought the other day?

Leyner: Original-recipe *Law & Order*, *Criminal Intent* (with SPECIAL VICTIMS UNIT ... which is reserved for the most HEINOUS crimes).

Leyner: *Triads in Love*?

Leyner: Excellent ... maybe you should get that for Jessica for Valentine's Day!

Gberg: That or a bath pillow.

Leyner: I bet I could pull a perfect 10 on the RigiScan ... thrown down a sick run on that RigiScan, dude.

Gberg: When the Leyner carnival comes to town, there is always a long line at the RigiScan.

Leyner: Nothing says I love you like a Mrs. Paul's frozen kidney pie and a chilled mango-calcium Propel.

Gberg: Love that new flavor.

Leyner: If you're having a romantic dinner at home, of course ... at Chez Goldberg.

Leyner: They didn't send me any of the calcium drinks ...

Gberg: I think I should e-mail the Propel folks before I answer the Gatorade and thirst question to get a quote.

Gberg: Or we can just regurgitate whatever they want us to say if it gets us more free stuff.

2:10 p.m.

Leyner: They sent me the poppy-flavored Propel with extra protein.

Gberg: I want to decorate my white coat at the hospital with Propel ads. Like a Nascar driver's jumpsuit.

Gberg: And get sprayed with the stuff when I make a good diagnosis.

Leyner: That's a cool idea ... doctors doing product placement!

Gberg: Don't think those bottom-feeding drug-company whores wouldn't try it.

Leyner: Y'all already walk around with your Viagra notepads and Lunesta panties?

Leyner: Isn't it interesting that the two most highly advertised drugs seem to be for getting erections AND falling asleep?????

Leyner: Talk about nocturnal tumescence.

Gberg: Right back to the RigiScan.

Leyner: A nice Viagra/sleeping pill cocktail ... and BANG ... instant nocturnal turgidity.

Gberg: I won't even use their stinkin' pens.

Gberg: I am a revolutionary. Like Che.

Gberg: And then postcoital blindness.

Leyner: Venceremos, or however you spell that.

Leyner: I think that's right!

Gberg: Yeah, preach, Brother Leyner, preach.

Is it true that you should eat a lot of carbohydrates the night before a marathon?

If you plan to run the New York City Marathon this year, you should reserve your Saturday night for the annual marathon eve dinner at Tavern on the Green. You can be sure that it will be a carbohydrate-heavy meal since its sponsor is a pasta company. Most marathons have similar meals, but these pre-event meals may not be entirely beneficial.

The old theory behind the big spaghetti meal was that carbohydrate loading could increase the glycogen in the muscles. Glycogen is stored carbohydrate in muscle and it serves as the body's reserve energy source. Fatigue during endurance activities is partially due to a depletion of muscle glycogen stores.

More recently, last-minute carbohydrate loading has been avoided by most serious marathoners. Experts believe that you should eat a normal diet with about 65 percent carbohydrates the week before the marathon. It is important not to increase your total calories.

If you eat a balanced meal the week before the marathon, you should have already loaded your body with glycogen, so there is no need to carry the extra weight from the big pasta meal. Also, it can be difficult to find a nice bathroom for a sit-down in New York City, and with a belly full of spaghetti bolognese you may need one somewhere around mile seventeen.

Will eating extra protein help build muscle mass?

If you have ever spent any time in Venice, California, or in Leyner's kitchen, you might have seen someone gorging himself on obscene amounts of egg whites prior to a workout.

Protein is a very important component of the diet, especially for athletes, but the amount of protein needed is often grossly overestimated. Eating tons of extra protein doesn't actually do much toward boosting your muscle mass and strength.

If your description of exercise is flipping channels with the remote and occasionally getting up to pee, then your protein needs are about 0.8 grams per kilogram of body weight. For a marathoner that number increases to 1.2 to 1.5 grams of protein per kilogram of body weight. If bodybuilding is your gig, you may need up to 1.8 to 2 grams per kilogram of body weight. The timing of protein intake is also important.

If you eat your egg whites with some carbohydrates within an hour after exercise, this combo stimulates the release of insulin and growth hormone. This leads to the growth of muscle.

What happens when you get the wind knocked out of you?

What happens? It's obvious. You gasp for air, feel like puking, whimper like a baby, and cry out for your mommy. The better question is, why?

The answer ... is that it's all about the diaphragm.

A blow to the gut, between the belly button and the heart, can cause a temporary paralysis of the diaphragm. This happens because this punch affects an area called the solar plexus, a dense cluster of nerve cells located behind the stomach just below the diaphragm. It is also known as the celiac plexus. When the diaphragm becomes paralyzed, you can't take in any air, hence the goldfish-flopping-on-the-kitchen-table feeling.

Does peeing in the shower cure athlete's foot?

Now wouldn't this be great! Finally, an excuse to pee in the shower.

Proponents of urine therapy claim that it is very

effective at eradicating athlete's foot. (Remember, some of these same people also suggest that drinking urine is good.) They may have a point, at least with the peeing on your foot. Urea, a major component of urine, is used in a cream to aid in the treatment of severe athlete's foot. Studies have shown that 40 percent urea cream increases the cure rate in athlete's foot when used with traditional antifungal creams. The urea cream doesn't exactly cure athlete's foot itself; it mostly serves to prepare and soften the tissue so that the antifungals can do their work.

So if you have a bad case of athlete's foot and insist on peeing on your feet, don't forget the fungal cream. Otherwise, all that shower peeing will be in vain.

Why do some people sweat excessively?

In doctor-speak, sweating is referred to as diaphoresis. Excessive sweating is called hyperhidrosis. When excessive sweating occurs in isolation with no apparent cause, it is called primary or essential hyperhidrosis. It is important to distinguish this condition from secondary hyperhidrosis, which can be associated with a variety of different conditions. These include tuberculosis, thyroid disease, tumors, reaction to medication, and menopause.

Primary hyperhidrosis can be focal (in one specific

area) or generalized. The most common areas affected are the palms and soles. This is called palmar-
plantar hyperhidrosis. You may also just get sweaty
pits, axillary hyperhidrosis, or facial sweating, craniofacial hyperhidrosis. Sweating may even occur excessively after an emotional outburst or eating spicy
food, called gustatory hyperhidrosis.

The cause of hyperhidrosis is unclear, though it is
present in almost 3 percent of the general population. There are many different treatments available,
from antiperspirants to surgery. Some medications
can prevent the stimulation of sweat glands, and
Botox has also been used successfully.

Can too much time on a bike lead to erectile dysfunction?

Studies have clearly shown that spending too much
time sitting on a bicycle seat can affect your "lift-off."
It's true, bike riders who spend a long time in the saddle are at greater risk of erectile dysfunction.

The problem here is that when you sit on a bicycle
seat, you put pressure on the perineum and on the
nerves and blood vessels that are responsible for
erectile function.

Anatomically, the perineum is the region between
the genital area and the anus.

Some of you may know the perineum by these
more exotic nicknames:

- nifkin.
- grundle.
- ABC (ass-ball connection).
- the runway.
- the no-fly zone.

Compression in this area leads to a decrease in penile blood flow and reduced oxygen in the area. This leads to penile fibrosis, which causes difficulty in the achievement of an erection. Gentlemen, choose your seat wisely. There is an increased prevalence of erectile dysfunction when using a narrow saddle.

Is it good or bad to masturbate/have sex the night before a big game?

"The trouble is not that players have sex the night before a game. It's that they stay out all night looking for it."

—Casey Stengel, baseball player and manager

This is definitely a topic that will capture an athlete's interest. A debate revolves around the myth that abstinence can improve an athlete's performance.

We know that testosterone levels fall temporarily after lovemaking. Testosterone allows humans to build muscle mass and strengthen performance, endurance, and physical ability. It also has been linked to aggression. Coaches who endorse a pre-event sexual abstinence policy believe that sexual frustration will increase aggression and that ejaculation of any kind will decrease testosterone.

Muhammad Ali was a strong proponent of the ejaculation embargo, and often went six weeks without any sexual satisfaction prior to a fight.

Ali was "The Greatest", but he probably could have forgone the embargo, without losing a fight. Scientific studies have never found a connection between abstinence and increased performance, endurance, or strength.

Bottom line—you can shoot and still score! Or score and still shoot!

Famous miler Marty Liquori had his own theory: "Sex makes you happy, and happy people don't run a mile in three minutes forty-seven seconds."

2:10 p.m.

Leyner: Nipple Brother ...

Leyner: I need to check a call that just came in ...

Leyner: Just in case it's Gaby's school ...

Gberg: Fancy LA call about your script?

Leyner: No ... just want to make sure a first-aid kit hasn't fallen on Gaby's head ... that once happened to her at school.

Gberg: That sucks, to get wounded by the first-aid kit.

Leyner: I'll be right back.

Gberg: I'll be waiting.

Leyner: OK.

Leyner: I'm back.

Gberg: And?

Gberg: Is it safe?

Leyner: Some telemarketer hawking a large-print scratch & sniff edition of *Why Do Men Have Nipples?*

Gberg: Perfect.

Leyner: Perfect.

Leyner: Let's take a lunchbreak, homie ... I'm so hungry.

2:20 p.m.

Gberg: Hey, I need something funny to add to "Is it good or bad to masturbate/have sex the night before a big game?" I found 2 great quotes from Casey Stengel and Marty Liquori.

Leyner: Need a burger and some curly fries.

Gberg: Also one from the *Rocky* movie where Mickey says, "Women weaken legs."

Leyner: I'll ponder it and come up with something, OK?

Gberg: Yeah, and let me know how your questions are coming.

Gberg: Go eat some meat.

Leyner: I bet Jack Johnson didn't adhere to that no-women-at-training-camp malarkey.

Gberg: Which Jack Johnson?

Leyner: The GREAT heavyweight champion!!

Gberg: The singer?

Leyner: NO!!!!!!!

Leyner: The singer probably masturbates before, during, and after "big games."

Gberg: Don't take such offense.

Leyner: I'm talking about Jack Johnson.

Leyner: OK ... sorry ... just a little hypersensitive when I get hungry.

Gberg: How dare I challenge your masculinity. Maybe you do fall asleep after sex.

Gberg: I fall asleep during.

2:25 p.m.

Leyner: I sleep with one eye open ...

Gberg: It's the Triad in you.

Is heading a soccer ball dangerous?

Some boxers are known to get a condition called dementia pugilistica from repeated punches to the head. This is also known as the punch-drunk syndrome or chronic traumatic encephalopathy, and it results from repeat concussions over many years. There is also some concern that heading a soccer ball could cause brain injury.

Head injury can definitely occur in soccer, but these injuries usually result from head-to-head rather than ball-to-head contact. There have been several studies that searched for the presence of injuries in competitive soccer players, and none has found a connection between ball-heading and brain injury. It is thought that the acceleration of the head caused by heading a soccer ball is not great enough to cause a concussion. There have been some advocates of soccer players wearing soft helmets, but these have not been found to reduce the risk of serious injury.

Why does the doctor say, "Turn your head and cough," when checking for a hernia?

First, a little lesson about hernias. (Welcome to hernia school!)

The general definition of a hernia is the protrusion of an organ or other bodily structure through the wall that normally contains it. There are many different types of hernias in the body, the most common of which is an inguinal hernia. This type of hernia occurs in the groin. There is an area in the groin called the inguinal canal. (Yes, it sounds a little bit like a vacation spot near Niagara Falls.) The inguinal canals are natural passages or openings through the muscles of the abdominal wall. They form a pathway for the testicles to descend from the abdomen into the scrotum. (This is not "The Flight of the Bumblebee" or *The Return of the Mummy* ... no, this is *The Descent of the*

Gonads.) Each canal usually closes before or right after birth. If this opening doesn't close, you may notice a lump in that region, or scrotal swelling. It could be your intestine that is poking through that hole. These hernias can either be congenital or acquired during adulthood. Inguinal hernias are more common in men than women.

Now, to the doctor … When the doctor is examining a patient for an inguinal hernia, he or she first tries to feel for the inguinal canal. For those of you who remember this part of the school sports physical, it's when you experience the frigid hand of some semiretired old doctor grasping your crotch. Coughing increases the pressure inside the abdomen. If you have a hernia or a defect in the inguinal canal, the increased pressure can push your intestine through the small hole and the doctor would feel this.

As for the "turn your head" part … this simply prevents you from coughing in the doctor's face.

Why do men need to wear a jock strap? (And why does it hurt so bad when you get kicked in the balls?)

The testicles are vulnerable little things, just hanging there in the scrotum with nothing protecting them from a vicious kick or punch. The testicles develop inside the abdomen and usually move down into the scrotum before birth. The nerves and blood vessels remain attached even as the testes descend. There is no muscle or bone to cushion a blow. Being covered in nerves adds to the unforgettable pain of getting kicked in the balls. That's why you feel it in the pit of your stomach when the vicious blow happens.

The jock strap or athletic supporter serves to support the testicles and keep them from flopping around, sort of like a sports bra for your balls. Most importantly, it can hold a hard plastic shell to protect you if you are participating in contact sports.

Do steroids shrink your testicles?

You may get big in some places on steroids, but it's true that other places might get smaller. Anabolic steroids or anabolic-androgenic steroids are synthetic derivatives of the male hormone testosterone. There are many side effects of short- and long-term use of these steroids. Male athletes who use anabolic steroids report increased sexual drive, aggression, acne, and increased body hair. Other attractive effects are reduced sperm count, impotence, breast development, and shrinking of the testicles. Steroid use can be extremely dangerous and can lead to premature heart attacks or strokes.

So if your intention in taking steroids is to look

like some sort of Herculean road warrior, remember—
you just may end up with man-boobs and micro-balls
instead.

• Chapter 4 •

No, I'm Not a Veterinarian!

We had just completed a long couples' session and after I had cleaned up the mess of ketchup and pudding that Leyner had smeared all over the walls, we strolled across the park to grab some lunch.

As we were about to cross the street, we noticed an elegantly accoutered woman hovering next to her defecating Doberman, her cupped hand engloved in a blue *New York Times* bag.

Leyner leaped to her side. "Let me get that for you," he offered gallantly and bare-handed the steaming poop, flinging it into a nearby trash receptacle.

The shocked woman gazed at Leyner with unmistakable affection. "That was remarkable. Bruno never lets anyone near his—" She blushed and averted her eyes. "His … movements. He's very sensitive about that. You have a way with animals, sir." She offered her hand for

Leyner to kiss. Leyner obliged and offered his. "I'll pass," she demurred.

She and the empty-boweled Bruno receded into the distance.

We then chanced upon, seated on a park bench, a man in his mid-fifties in a frayed thrift-store suit playing chess with a more impeccably dressed chimpanzee, attired in a freshly pressed white shirt and a red bow tie.

We quietly ate our lunch, our eyes riveted to the game of chess, which, from my limited knowledge of the game, was being played at an extremely high level.

The man had opened with the classic Ruy Lopez— white king's pawn to king four, etc., etc., etc. Soon he had control over the center of the board and had placed the chimp's black queen in a desperately untenable position. The chimp seemed baffled by his predicament, when he noticed Leyner staring him down. He leaped from his seat, rushed toward Leyner, and began to furiously and frantically pick at the hairs on the back of Leyner's neck.

Leyner embraced the chimp, groomed him with reciprocal affection, and whispered something into his new friend's ear.

The chimp bounced off Leyner's lap, returned to the board, and began a focused series of tactically brilliant moves that soon left the man no choice but to resign in stunned and abject defeat.

Putting his iPod headphones back on and cranking up Salt-N-Pepa's "Push It," the chimp turned toward Leyner and proudly pumped a victorious fist in the air.

Leyner stood and silently saluted his simian soul mate.

"Leyner ... I'm impressed ... I've never seen this side of you before ... You're like Dr. Friggin' Doolittle," I said.

Leyner acknowledged the compliment with a modest bow of the head. And we returned to the office.

Do animals commit suicide?

Heaven knows, animals would be completely justified in becoming suicidally depressed. There's the brutal hierarchy of the food chain out there on the savannah, and the benumbing life of captivity in some squalid zoo where junior-high-school jocks toss spicy snacks and laxatives into your cage, or having some goofy owner who insists on dressing you in a little patterned doggie vest. It's all more than enough to make even the perkiest Pollyanna in the animal kingdom want to blow his brains out. But animals don't really commit suicide, at least not in the way we humans define the term.

Lemmings have traditionally been the poster boys for suicidal animals. But they aren't as self-destructive as they seem. Lemmings sometimes fall off cliffs during mass migration, but these deaths are accidental rather than intentional. There are several other examples of animals who appear to commit suicide. There's the mother octopus feeding its young, but not herself. And the Australian crab spider, which produces a special batch of eggs too jumbo to be laid—so her hatched spiderlings actually gnaw into her body to consume them, eventually killing poor ol' Mom. Both of these examples are open to anthropomorphic misinterpretation, but don't seem to represent suicide as we know it.

Although animals are known to mope, they have never been observed locking themselves in their bedrooms with the blinds drawn, and listening to morose, self-pitying dirges by Leonard Cohen or The Cure for hours on end.

Do dogs have belly buttons?

Dogs are placental mammals and therefore they do have a belly button. That does not make it easy to find. It is there somewhere in all that fur about halfway between the rib cage and the hip bone. While you are looking, feel free to give Rover a little scratch, but watch out for the shaking leg.

Can a cockroach get stuck in my ear?

Remember when you were told not to put anything bigger than your elbow in your ear? The roaches weren't listening. It is not uncommon to see patients in the emergency room with cockroaches in their ears. The cockroaches have an easy time crawling in, but they aren't very good at backing out. A moving cockroach in your external ear causes great pain and anxiety. In the ER, we first put mineral oil or Lidocaine (an anesthetic liquid) in the ear to suffocate the trespassing creature. We then employ an "alligator forceps"—a long, thin tweezer-like instrument to pull the intruder out.

How do we know that dogs are colorblind?

I imagine it would be very difficult to get the dog to sit still at the eye doctor long enough to find out. So how do we know that dogs are colorblind?

To begin with, they aren't. They don't see as many colors as humans, but they do see more than black and white. Dogs have two types of cells on their retina that recognize wavelengths of light, called cones. Humans have three types of cones, so we see more colors. It is likely that dogs confuse reds and greens. This type of vision is similar to humans who are red-green colorblind.

How do we know?

Scientists taught dogs to recognize colors, but they often confused reds and greens. Beams of light were also flashed into dogs' eyes and the pattern of light that was reflected back was analyzed. These results were then compared with the pattern produced when the same lights were flashed into human eyes.

What does a chimpanzee do with the umbilical cord after it has a baby?

Bites it … and probably eats it. Many species of wild mammals (primates, and thus chimps included) conveniently chow down on the umbilical cord, and also eat their placenta. One good reason, in addition to the irresistible availability of a highly nutritious meal, is that quickly disposing of the umbilical cord and placenta protects the newborn offspring from predators that might be attracted to the bloody organs. As far as we *Homo sapiens* go, there are rare (excuse the choice of words) instances of placentophagy (placenta eating) in human society—notwithstanding persistent urban-myth-like tales of pervasive "placenta parties" thrown by hippie earth mothers during the 1970s in—where else?—California. Most cultures have specific and strict taboos against this postpartum entree. And that's probably, as the doyenne of fine dining and all things domestic—Martha Stewart—would say: a good thing.

Do toads cause warts?

Poor, poor toads. They seem to always take a back seat to frogs. Frogs get kissed and turn into princes, and toads just get to cause warts. Well, here is some good news for toads. Toads do not cause warts. Toads do, however, produce a substance from the parotid gland behind the eyes to act as protection. This toxin can make other animals very sick if ingested and can be irritating to the eyes. Some people even go way beyond touching toads and will lick them in an attempt to get high from a supposed psychedelic substance on their skin.

A special type of toad, the Bufo toad, does contain a psychedelic substance, but it doesn't cause hallucinations. Be careful, because people have been arrested for toad licking.

Are bulls really attracted to the color red?

What would a bullfight be without the red cape? Answer: a bullfight just the same. However, a yellow cape might be more easily stained with blood. Bulls probably do react to a bright color but not specifically to red. The movement of the cape is more key to catching the bull's attention.

Why don't vultures get sick from eating rotten meat?

You'd think chowing down on rotten carcasses of putrefying, maggot-ridden meat might not be the best thing for a bird (never mind the bad breath it causes). But it doesn't seem to bother vultures, who dine al fresco on the stuff whenever they get the chance. Granted, they prefer their carrion (that's dead flesh, not luggage) to be fresh, not festering— although they're not terribly picky. But vultures do not get sick from eating rotten or diseased meat, even if the dead animal being scarfed down is infected with botulism, cholera, or anthrax. Talk about having a strong stomach! Disease organisms just don't survive in a vulture's digestive tract. And that's not true for other carrion-junkies like hyenas and jackals. Although vultures have an extremely high acid level in their bellies, it's not known precisely what kills off all the nasty pathogens in this big bird's iron gut.

(Health Advisory: If you're feeling especially listless and rundown, and you find that, whenever you step outside, vultures are wheeling over your head, licking their chops, they may know something you don't know. See a doctor.)

Is a dog's mouth clean?

Joel Leyner propounded two axiomatic truths for the entirety of his son Mark's childhood: 1. Someday every single person will possess his or her own helicopter and commute to work in it; and 2. A dog's mouth is actually cleaner than a person's. Well, so much for fatherly wisdom. Although Leyner never really bought the helicopter prediction—seemed like too much of a rush-hour nightmare—the dog's mouth assertion seemed plausible. But the ol' man was wrong on that score too. When the oral cultures from ten randomly chosen people were compared with samples from the mouths of ten randomly chosen hounds, guess what? The "yuck factor"—that is, bacterial colonies per square centimeter—was greater in the majority of mutt mouths than in the person pie-holes. No wonder Lucy hated it when Snoopy kissed her.

5:16 p.m.

Gberg: What's up, Nipple Brother?

Leyner: Working on a section for our calendar called "Life After Death or Maggot Chow."

Gberg: I am trying to get some work done on book #2.

Gberg: The "B" side of our literary record.

Leyner: Hold on ...

Gberg: We used to feed our dog maggot chow.

Leyner: That's funny ... wait, I'm finishing this thing ...

5:20 p.m.

Gberg: I am doing some research for the book. Did I tell you that Carrie wants the book earlier if possible?

Leyner: We all agreed on March 1.

5:25 p.m.

Gberg: She said if possible.

Leyner: Tell her to stick her head in an autoclave.

Gberg: Absolutely.

Leyner: Well, all right then.

Do rats cause rabies?

Rats have such an undeservedly bad image. Rats are rarely, if ever, infected with rabies, and have never been known to cause rabies among humans in the United States. Woodchucks are far more prone to be infected than rats, and raccoons are the most common wild animals to have rabies. As far as the transmission of human rabies is concerned, bats have been responsible for almost 75 percent of rabies cases since 1990.

So let's lighten up on the rats, okay? It's so unfair. People are still blaming rats for the Black Death (the bubonic plague epidemic that killed 20 million people in fourteenth-century Europe), when it was actually the fleas' that lived on the rats fault (*Xenopsylla cheopis*, to be exact).

In an effort to rehabilitate the reputation of the rat, here's a list of our favorite rat songs:

"Eat That Rat" by the Ramones
"Rats" by Pearl Jam
"Rats in the Cellar" by Aerosmith
Anything by the bands Ratt or the Boomtown Rats
And, of course, the GREATEST rat song ever: "Ben" by Michael
  Jackson

Why do people say, "I need to piss like a horse"?

A horse is a pretty big animal, and it's a good rule of thumb (or rule of bladder) that the bigger the animal, the bigger the bladder, which means the bigger the puddle. In adult humans, the average urine production is one to two liters per day. Normal urination for a 1,000-pound horse is about one to two gallons a day. And then there's the horse's famously forceful urinary stream—a torrent that could blast rioting demonstrators against a wall!

But this saying may actually have gained currency as the result of the widespread practice of giving racehorses a drug called furosemide prior to a race. Ostensibly a preventive measure for exercise-induced pulmonary hemorrhaging (EPIH), the drug has also been found to have a clear performance-enhancing effect. Why? Probably because furosemide is a diuretic—it makes you piss—and horses given furosemide lose about twenty pounds of their pre-race body weight through urination. And, at the track, lighter means faster.

Horses, by the way, aren't the only animals in sports subject to chemical cheating. Police in Shanghai, China, recently shut down a gambling den where fighting crickets were given performance-enhancing drugs!

For the hauntingly poetic qualities of horse piss, check out the renowned seventeenth-century

Japanese haiku master Matsuo Basho, who wrote the following poem (which appears in his collection *Narrow Road to the Deep North*):

> *Bitten by fleas and lice,*
> *I slept in a bed,*
> *a horse pissing all the time by my pillow.*

Okay, maybe it loses a little something in the translation.

Why don't mosquito bites hurt when you get them, and why do they itch?

Ahh ... the amazing, diabolically ingenious mosquito. A mosquito stabs you with its piercing-sucking pro-boscis, which is actually made up of several needle-like tubes. She (only the females bite) then injects you with her saliva laced not only with an anticoagulant, so your blood won't clot and can flow easily up her tiny straw, but also an anesthetic, so you won't feel the pain and whack the little bugger in the midst of its vampiric Happy Meal. The itching you feel later on is an immune response to the foreign proteins in the saliva left behind in the wound.

Try to resist the almost irresistible urge to scratch your mosquito bites. It'll only make the itching worse, and could even lead to infection. Calamine lotion is a better bet. That dappled-with-blobs-of-pink-gook look won't garner much kudos on the fashion run-way, but at least you'll feel better.

Leyner, who fancies himself something of an amateur entomologist, is particularly obsessed with mosquitoes. Here, from the pages of *Travel & Leisure* magazine, is his lovely description of the large mos-quitoes that inhabit the Canadian Arctic province of Nunavut in the warmer summer months: "The mos-quitoes here are enormous and ravenous. They actu-ally gaze up at you while sucking, like in a porn movie."

Why are some people sweeter to mosquitoes?

There are many different factors and variables that come into play when a mosquito chooses to bite you over someone else or vice versa. So don't take it per-sonally either way. The carbon dioxide released when we exhale is an extremely important attractant, as is the lactic acid produced by muscle movement, as is moist skin and a warm body. Sebum, eccrine, and apocrine secretions—basically, sweat—are also major chemo-attractants for these annoying creatures. And mosquitoes have a yen for heavily scented grooming products—particularly floral fragrances in perfumes, aftershaves, soaps, lotions, and hair-care products.

Short of not emitting carbon dioxide, lactic acid, or heat—in other words, not moving or breathing, which might also mean you're dead—the only way you ensure that you're "sour" to a mosquito is probably to use repellent.

Why are bugs attracted to light?

Phototaxis is an organism's automatic movement toward or away from light. Cockroaches are negatively phototactic. Turn on that kitchen light and off they scurry to their dark little holes. But many insects are positively phototactic—as evidenced by the mass bug graves in your light fixtures. Many people are also phototactic, especially for the "limelight"—those of us who secretly crave the strobe fusillade of paparazzi flashbulbs and murmur, "Mr. DeMille, I'm ready for my close-up," in our dreams … But, back to bugs. There are a variety of reasons that various insects are positively phototactic. Many insects, including bees, orient themselves in relation to the sun. Certain nocturnal bugs—moths, for instance—use moonlight to navigate, flying at a certain angle to the moon's light rays to maintain a straight trajectory. When it approaches a source closer than the moon—say, a light bulb—a moth perceives the light as stronger in one eye than the other, causing one wing to beat faster, so it flies in a tightening spiral, ever closer to the light. Some bugs are sensitive to ultraviolet light reflected by flowers at night. Artificial lights that emit UV rays will also be attractive to these guys. Other bugs are drawn to the heat that incandescent bulbs produce at night. Fireflies are bugs and bulbs all in one. They use their bioluminescence to attract each other.

Do bees die after they sting you?

Only honeybees die after stinging, but not bumble-bees or wasps. A honeybee's barbed stinger is actual-ly attached to its abdomen. When this stinger lodges in the flesh, and the bee tries to escape, the stinger is ripped from its body, tearing off most of the bee's belly (along with a nerve ganglion, various muscles, a venom sac, and the end of its digestive tract), and the bee dies of the injuries.

Although the self-inflicted fatality of the honey-bee's sting lacks the individual consciousness and premeditation to truly be considered kamikaze-like, you still have to admire that take-one-for-the-hive esprit de corps.

And research also indicates that it's only in old car-toons that bees chase you around the countryside, their swarm taking the shape of a harpoon or large pub dart.

Is it true that sharks have to keep swimming to stay alive?

Sharks do not have "swim bladders"—the gas-filled balloon-like organ that enable most fish to stay afloat and upright in water. This means that, since a shark's body is heavier than water, it will indeed sink when not swimming. Some sharks, including great whites and hammerheads, actually have to keep swimming to breathe. They need to constantly move forward in order to pass oxygen-bearing water over their gills— a process called obligate ramjet ventilation. But there are many species of shark that do not have to swim to breathe. Other common misconceptions about sharks are that they don't have eyelids and never sleep. Fish have no eyelids, but sharks actually have elaborate eyelids and some even have an additional, protective eyelid called a nictitating membrane. There is some debate among marine biologists as to whether sharks actually sleep or not, but most think that sharks do slow down their brain functions from time to time and go on a sort of "autopilot." In fact, sharks may swim in their "sleep," although it's not the sort of snoring, drooling, butt-scratching snooze we're accustomed to.

Why do dogs wag their tails?

Most people think that dogs wag their tails only when they're happy. But it's a little more complicated than that. Canine tail-wagging is a form of communication (dogs don't usually wag their tails when they're alone), but it can relate a variety of emotional states, as anyone who's been bitten by a tail-wagging dog knows full well. The wag can convey good spirits, fear, aggression, dominance, or submission. The well-known zoologist Desmond Morris contends that a dog's wagging tail expresses a state of conflict—the simultaneous need to advance and retreat. Some have suggested that tail wagging is simply a physiological means of getting rid of surplus energy. P. Dwight Tapp, who's conducted research at the University of Toronto in the cognitive functions and brain structures of dogs, points out that wagging also spreads pheromones by causing the muscles around the anus to contract, pressing on glands that release a scent. This scent communicates information about sex, age, and social status to other dogs.

There's another compelling question about canine behavior: Why don't dogs, whose loathsome, irresponsible owners leave them tethered to parking meters in dangerously frigid temperatures and then spend several hours leisurely browsing in Walmart, rip their faces off (or at least viciously maul them) when they finally come out, instead of enthusiastically wagging their tails?

Is it true that cockroaches can survive an atomic blast?

The poor, loathsome, reviled cockroach, persona non grata wherever it goes, chased from one corner of the earth to the other by brandished shoes and rolled-up magazines … But you gotta give the vermin their due, because, yes, they could probably withstand the radiation in a thermonuclear blast. A human being exposed to radiation in excess of about 800 rems (the "rem" is a dosage of radiation that will cause a specific amount of harm to human tissue) will most likely die. The killer dose for an American cockroach is 67,500 rems. And a German cockroach would need to be nuked with about 100,000 rems to stop it in its tracks! There's a simple reason cockroaches (along with other insects) are less vulnerable to radiation than humans—their simplicity. The more complex and longer living an organism is, the more vulnerable it is to the effects of radiation, i.e. the more there is to go wrong. And cockroaches don't live long enough to develop the cancers associated with radiation exposure.

Researchers at Stanford University are actually designing and building robots based on cockroaches—not because they're nuke-proof, but because they're so speedy and agile. (Some cockroaches can move fifty times their body length in one second. That's about the equivalent of a human being running at 200 miles per hour!)

If all this has whetted your intellectual appetite for cockroaches, W. J. Bell's *The Laboratory Cockroach* is a *must-read*. It includes such essential information as "How to Anesthetize a Cockroach" and, of course, "How to Extract the Sex Pheromone of a Cockroach." (Who knows when THAT might come in handy?)

Cockroaches haven't evolved much in the millions of years they've been around, and they'll probably be scurrying about for zillions to come. And would you really want to live in a post-nuclear apocalyptic wasteland populated only by mutant Madagascar hissing cockroaches? Probably not. But what if you could hunker down and survive somehow … and you'd be the only human alive … and the cockroaches would worship you as some sort of god? Hmmmmm …

Can animals be gay?

Yes they can! According to biologist Bruce Bagemihl, there is documented evidence that some 450 species engage in "gay" and "lesbian" sexual activity, including whiptail lizards, bottlenose dolphins, flamingoes, vampire bats, giraffes, and penguins. According to a recent study on sheep, published in the journal *Endocrinology*, approximately 8 percent of rams exhibit sexual preferences for other male partners, instead of for ewes. Then, of course, you've got your bonobos—those scandalously hedonistic, orgiastic, no-holds-barred sensualists of the ape world—that do it all: heterosexual, homosexual, bisexual, bondage, golden showers, leather, rubber, enemas, you name it. Earthworms, tapeworms, leeches, and snails are hermaphrodites, in case you're into that sort of thing. We've yet to come upon a case of cross-species identity disorder—for instance, a platypus that feels it's actually a kinkajou but born in a platypus's body.

Do animals masturbate?

Yes, animals masturbate, as anyone with a leg that has been vigorously humped by a randy Jack Russell terrier will readily attest. (I know, humping may also be a form of play and an expression of dominance, but it's obviously sexual, and some dogs have orgasms doing it, so let's be real about it.)

According to Professor Keith Kendrik, head of the Neurobiology Programme and Laboratory of Cognitive and Developmental Neuroscience at the Barraham Institute at Cambridge University, many male mammals touch and lick themselves to achieve erection, but only in primates is masturbation to ejaculation observed. Colobus, talapoins, macaques, baboons, mangabeys, mandrills, orangutans, gorillas, and chimpanzees, you know who you are … Female mammals, and especially female primates, have also been seen masturbating. (It does sounds a little kinky, watching them like that, but it's science, and some-body's gotta do it.) In fact, as a team of scientists writing in the journal *Science* recently concluded after observing orangutans in Borneo and Sumatra, the resourceful apes had learned the art of masturbating with sticks.

As long as we're talking about animal sexuality, you may be interested to know which creature is the most well-endowed in the world. Without a doubt, the blue whale is the Tommy Lee of the animal king-dom—its penis is eleven feet long, and its testicles weigh up to a hundred pounds each. Another inter-esting fact is that Aristotle Onassis is said to have upholstered the bar stools on his yacht *Christina* with whale-penis leather. (If this sort of stuff intrigues you, you might find it worth your while, next time you're in Reykjavik, to visit the Icelandic Phallological Museum. It is devoted entirely to the study of animal penises and houses ninety-nine specimens.)

If you intend to go online and do your own ama-teur research on animal masturbation or penis leather, be forewarned. You will inadvertently sum-mon up a witch's brew of extremely disturbing websites.

Do some people really have tails?

If you saw the movie *Shallow Hal*, you might remember Jason Alexander's (George from *Seinfeld*) character with his small, wagging tail. This is another example of how you can't believe everything that you see in the movies.

This doesn't mean that people can't have tails. It's just that they can't wag them. Human tails or dorsal cutaneous appendages are rare congenital defects. These "tails" have none of the characteristics of true animal tails. True tails contain bones or have associated muscles that permit movement. The human tail is usually just a fatty outgrowth of skin right at the base of the spine, and often a sign that there might be an underlying spinal defect.

2:03 p.m.

Gberg: Jefe. *¿Que pasa?*

Gberg: I am Jefe, you are Uno. Sorry.

Leyner: Help!!

Gberg: What?

Leyner: I love this research!!

Gberg: How was the Dublin interview, you lusty leprechaun?

Leyner: Do you know there's an Icelandic Phallological Museum in Reykjavik?

2:05 p.m.

Gberg: I'll meet you at JFK!

Gberg: Or is Newark easier for you?

Leyner: We need to put an animal penis size q. in the vet. chapter ... or I'll just add some stuff to the gay animal q. & a.

Gberg: I spent hours last night on the sun sneezing question. I still can't believe that there is science behind that.

Leyner: Aristotle Onassis had his bar stools on his yacht *Christina* covered in whale-penis leather.

Gberg: Poor whale.

Leyner: I want whale-penis leather pants.

Gberg: You could wear that to your cable TV interview. Then you might pass the dress code.

Leyner: Just think how I'd look in those next time we're on *The Today Show*??

Leyner: I know, right?

Gberg: I can just hear the narration as you stroll down the red carpet. Leyner looks marvelous in his Moby-Dicks!

Leyner: I'd wear my whale-penis leather pants and a nice, simple hummingbird-wing blouse.

Leyner: Moby-Dicks!!!!

Leyner: The new "Calvins."

Gberg: That would be a great final competition for *Project Runway*.

Leyner: Hey, I have a medical problem ... give me IM advice, Mr. Man.

2:10 p.m.

Gberg: Each of you has been given one whale penis and 100 dollars ...

Leyner: I think I have a splinter in my BIG TOE ... and it's SO FUCKING PAINFUL ... I can't walk on it at all ... but it's not sticking out so I can't grab it with my trusty tweezers ... what's a Nipple Brother to do???

Gberg: Are you sure it's not infected? Unusual to be so painful. I could remove it if you wanted to come over.

Gberg: I have some rusty tools that would be perfect for you.

Leyner: Rusty tools ... I'm drooling with anticipation.

Leyner: Don't know if it's infected ... just looks like there's a little dark fragment in there ... but it hurts so much to put any weight on it ... otherwise it doesn't hurt.

2:15 p.m.

Leyner: Anyway ... I should get back to researching.

Leyner: Should I soak my toe for a while and try to get the thing out ...? Does soaking work?

Gberg: Soaking is good.

Gberg: Use Buddy Ebsen salts.

Leyner: Sorry ... I've been at this researching thing since 9 and I'm a little off my game.

Gberg: I actually have no idea what epsom salts are.

Leyner: OK … thanks, Jefe. What are you up to for the rest of the day?

Leyner: I'll use kosher salt, thank you very much.

Gberg: I need to go do some work on the book. I will call you later.

Leyner: Don't know what that is either.

Leyner: Talk to you later.

Gberg: Ciao.

Chapter 5

Insemination, Gestation, and Lactation (the Preggers Chapter)

I had kept our next patient away from Leyner on her last two visits. Isabel Collier, thirty-two years old and twenty-two weeks pregnant, was not in the right hormonal state to deal with Leyner's unorthodox therapeutic style. She had come to see me to address her fears about becoming a parent. Her husband was unavailable for the earlier sessions, but had accompanied her today. I thought perhaps the support of her husband would allow a smooth transition for Leyner's introduction.

We were seated in the office when Wendy Thurston brought the loving couple through the door. Leyner immediately jumped to his feet, clapping his hands with blithe, almost childlike enthusiasm.

I motioned for the couple to sit down and immediately tears of shame began rolling down the expectant mother's full face.

"I can't do this … I can't. I'm not prepared to raise a child. I'm so ashamed to admit this … " She turned to her husband entreatingly. "Please forgive me," she wept.

The husband embraced her and was about to begin reassuring her, when he looked up and began sniffing the air.

"Did somebody crap their pants?" he asked, grimacing.

"I made a poop," Leyner announced, beaming.

"You what?" replied the husband. "What kind of sick freaking place is this?"

I wondered the same thing, but realized that Leyner might have stumbled onto something.

"Please, I know this seems unusual, but Leyner is trying to show you something."

"It's yucky poopy," Leyner whined, squirming in his seat.

"Honey, go help him," the wife said, nudging her husband and wiping her eyes.

"Me? I didn't come here to wipe a grown man's ass!"

Leyner looked up at him with big, sad eyes, pouting. "Daddy?"

Off went the husband and Leyner to the men's room.

I turned to the wife. "My partner is unusual, but a true genius. Let's just hope they don't get into a fistfight."

Moments later, the husband returned carrying Leyner in his arms. Leyner was covered head to toe with baby powder, and the two men were engaged in a spirited discussion about the ergonomics of different strollers.

As I began to explore a range of issues concerning the woman's anxiety about her impending maternity, Leyner began tossing a ball to the husband. He began winging it harder and harder until the husband responded with a ninety-mile-an-hour hummer directed at Leyner's head. The ball sailed through the open window out onto the street. Leyner leaped through the window as Isabel stood and berated her husband.

"How many times have I told you not to play ball in the house. It sets a bad example. Look what you've done!"

I interrupted. "Very good. You are setting boundaries and cooperatively parenting. You two are naturals."

At that, there was a knock at the door. Leyner re-entered, arm in arm with a tall, buxom Swedish woman. He looked at his surrogate parents and said, "This is Inga. We met on an exchange program. We're engaged!" he squealed.

I looked at the woman again and noticed very large hands and a trace of a five o'clock shadow.

I could see the husband also giving the "girlfriend" a skeptical once-over.

He leaned toward his wife and whispered, "I think it's a guy, for Christ sake."

"Honey … look how happy he is," the wife responded, squeezing her husband's hand with affectionate pride.

"Happy? He's engaged to Arnold Schwarzenegger!"

The woman stood and tenderly took one of Leyner's hands and grabbed one of the meaty paws of the fiancé. "Sweetheart, if the two of you are happy, we're happy." They all embraced.

"Do you see what you just did?" I asked. "Acceptance is a sign of unconditional love. I'm proud of both of you. You've shown in one session a remarkable capacity to deal with each phase of your child's dependence, maturation, and separation."

The woman had a look of absolute bliss on her face. "We did, didn't we?"

She looked proudly at her husband.

"Let's go celebrate, I have an overwhelming craving for kielbasa sausage."

"I know just the place," said Leyner, as the two couples sauntered out through the door.

I was left alone in the office to ponder the complexities of pregnancy and parenting. I also wondered why I ever left the ER and got mixed up with this strange little man.

Does standing on your head after sex increase your chances of becoming pregnant?

Getting pregnant can be a tricky business for some. As couples are trying to conceive at older ages, the process has become more regimented, mechanical, and scientific. Temperatures are taken, ovulation kits are scattered across the bedroom, and books are piled on the bedside table. It's a miracle that there is even time for sex. Once the sex finally happens, the postcoital positioning begins. Some experts believe that lying down for twenty to thirty minutes after sex may boost your chances of conceiving. Others recommend a pillow placed under the hips to add a little gravity to the mix.

There is no evidence to suggest that standing on your head will help at all, although it would be very interesting to try. If you don't conceive, you could at least get a job with Cirque du Soleil.

Should a man wait several days between sex to store up sperm if trying to impregnate his wife?

Having to go give a sample for semen analysis can be a strange experience. I (Dr. Billy) would be happy to share my own story. Typically, when you go to the doctor to give a semen specimen, you're sent to a small room with magazines and videos to help you along. When you finish your business, you place it in a door in the wall and off you go. I experienced several problems during this process. One difficulty was how long I needed to wait before giving them the sample. The process doesn't really take *that* long, but isn't it more respectable to wait awhile to, y'know, show some stamina? Then there's the disappointment when you finally look at the end product. They will be measuring not only the quality, but also the quantity, and the amount can look pretty paltry. I left that day feeling dejected, as if I'd just failed an important test. Alas, the results were very good and I was able to do a little victory dance in the office when the results came in. (That would be my Viable Sperm Dance, not to be confused with the Funky Chicken.)

If you have to provide a sample for semen analysis, doctors ask you to abstain from ejaculation for two to five days. But this doesn't necessarily mean that abstention is good for improving the odds of conception.

Studies agree that semen volume and sperm concentration increase with prolonged sexual abstinence. The issue of sperm motility is different. Sperm motility is believed to be one of the most important parameters in evaluating fertilizing ability. The percentage of normal sperm and the percentage of motile sperm decrease with infrequent ejaculation. Overall, studies find that ejaculating several times per week will give you the highest number of fully functional sperm.

Are more babies conceived during a full moon?

It is not uncommon to hear this myth in the hospital. People seem to firmly believe that more babies are conceived when the moon is full and that more are born when the moon is full. Studies show absolutely no correlation between the moon and pregnancy. This is another one of those old wives' tales that people just don't want to relinquish.

In 2005, in an article appearing in the *American Journal of Obstetrics and Gynecology* entitled "Birth Rate and Its Correlation with the Lunar Cycle and Specific Atmospheric Conditions," a group of doctors in Arizona once again tested this idea and found no correlation.

Can a woman get pregnant from pre-ejaculation?

Pre-ejaculate has many other names including Cowper's fluid, pre-come, pre-cum, and speed drop. It is secreted by Cowper's glands, and it serves to lubricate the urethra and prepare it for the passage of sperm.

Studies have shown that pre-ejaculatory fluid does not contain sperm and therefore cannot be responsible for pregnancies. Although there is no sperm in pre-come itself, there could be some residual sperm in the urethra from a recent sexual encounter or ejaculation. Therefore, there is the risk of pregnancy with any intercourse.

Diseases can also be transferred in pre-ejaculate, so don't fall for that old line "I will just put it in for a second so you can see how it feels."

Why do you have a "bionic" sense of smell when you are pregnant?

The journal *Chemical Senses* isn't usually at the top of my reading list, but it certainly came in handy to answer this question. In 2004, it published an article entitled "A Longitudinal Descriptive Study of Self-Reported Abnormal Smell and Taste Perception in Pregnant Women." The article described the "odor hedonics" of pregnancy. Say what? I love it when they use fancy terms instead of just saying the perception of pleasant or unpleasant smells in pregnancy.

This article and others confirm the idea that pregnant women have an especially acute sense of smell. This is more common in early pregnancy and disappears after delivery. These authors go on to speculate that the abnormalities in smell may be explained by some natural internal mechanism to avoid poisons. They noted that the odors of cigarette smoke, alcohol, and coffee in particular were commonly reported as being perceived as stronger than normal during early pregnancy.

It is postulated that this bionic sense of smell is caused by an increase in hormones, specifically plasma estradiol (an estrogen). Women also have an increase in estradiol during the menstrual cycle, with a peak at ovulation (around day fourteen). Some women report increased sense of smell during this period of their cycle as well.

Whatever the reason or cause, I have found the bionic sense of smell very troublesome. During my own wife's pregnancy, I was forced to shower immediately upon entering the house, loofah myself aggressively with a rough sea sponge, brush my teeth excessively, and scrape my tongue with barbaric oral-hygiene implements … And despite my best efforts, I was still occasionally put outside like a bag of rotten garbage.

Why can't you eat soft cheese during pregnancy?

So pickles and ice cream are okay, but soft cheese is a problem? That doesn't seem to make a great deal of sense, does it? It's really all about *Listeria monocytogenes*. This bacterium is found in raw, unpasteurized milk and any cheeses or other dairy products made from it. It can cause a potentially deadly disease called listeriosis.

Listeriosis usually isn't a big problem in healthy individuals, but pregnancy makes you more vulnerable. This bacteria is about seventeen times more likely to cause an infection in pregnant women than in the normal population. Listeriosis usually only causes mild "flu-like" symptoms, but the real problem lies in the fact that it can be transferred across the placenta and harm the baby. Listeria during pregnancy can cause miscarriage, premature rupture of membranes, premature birth, and very serious infections in newborns including meningitis.

But don't freak out if you are pregnant and mistakenly chow down some fresh mozzarella. Listeriosis is relatively rare.

Do any of these things induce labor: sex, spicy food, Chinese food, red wine?

Here are the makings for a romantic evening of freedom before the baby's arrival: a spicy Szechuan meal, a nice glass of cabernet, and some sweet lovemaking. The good news is that you can repeat it several times because it will probably not induce labor. There is no science behind the myth that spicy food, Chinese food, red wine, eggplant, or castor oil can bring baby sooner.

Sex is another issue. Semen contains a high concentration of prostaglandins, and prostaglandins are often used for cervical ripening and induction of labor. Nipple stimulation during sex can also cause contractions and may help bring on labor if the cervix is already ripe. Husbands, inducing labor this way may be hard work, but—hey—somebody's gotta do it.

Is it true that when you put your arms up when you are pregnant, the umbilical cord wraps around the baby's neck?

I get anxious every time the subject of an umbilical cord around the neck comes up. I flash back to an emergency delivery that I had to do in an elevator at the hospital back when I was a resident. A patient came into the ER who was about to deliver, but we thought there was time enough to get her upstairs to labor and delivery. So, accompanied by a nursing student and a "BOA kit" (Baby-on-Arrival kit), up we went. While entering the elevator, the woman pointed between her legs and said in Spanish, "*El bebe, el bebe.*" With the elevator doors closing, I had to do the delivery right there, but the cord was wrapped tightly around the baby's neck. I was able to get the cord over the baby's head, but the baby was a little blue when it came out. The BOA kit comes with a bulb syringe to clean out the baby's nose and mouth, but the frantic nursing student had ripped it open and the bulb syringe had fallen on the floor. Luckily, by the time she finally found the syringe, the baby had turned a healthy pink and let go with a reassuringly robust cry. When the elevator doors finally opened, the poor nursing student went crying to the ER, and I was left to be mocked by the labor and delivery nurses for arriving in such a frantic state.

In approximately 20 percent of all births, the cord is wrapped around the baby's neck. This is called a nuchal cord and usually causes no problems. A nuchal cord is caused by fetal movements. It certainly has nothing to do with anything that the mother has done, especially her arm movements. So, pregnant ladies, in the words of Grandmaster Flash, "Throw your hands in the air! And wave 'em like you just don't care!"

Is there any surefire way to determine the sex of the baby?

There is a very long list of mythical methods for determining the sex of your unborn child, such as:

- More fetal kicking indicates a boy.
- More early-pregnancy morning sickness indicates a girl.
- Sexual position at conception can affect whether you have a male or female child.

- If the fetal heart rate is fast, you will have a boy; if it's slow, a girl.
- Carrying high, it will be a boy, carrying low, a girl.
- Using the Chinese lunar calendar to determine sex.
- Hold a wedding ring on a string—if it moves like a pendulum, a boy; if it spins in a circle, a girl.

Unfortunately, none of these old wives' tales have been scientifically validated. If you want certainty, you need an amniocentesis. Modern ultrasound can also determine fetal sex.

The sex of the baby is determined at conception, and we have no control over choosing the sex at that moment either. The father can actually take credit for the gender as the sex of your baby is determined by the dad's sperm. If sperm carrying an X-chromosome fertilizes the egg, the baby will be a girl, and if sperm carrying a Y-chromosome fertilizes the egg, you will be the parent of a boy.

Can you breast-feed with fake boobs?

In 2004, approximately 334,000 breast augmentations were performed, according to the American Society for Aesthetic Plastic Surgery (ASAPS). The largest percentage of breast augmentation surgeries occur in women between the ages of nineteen and thirty-four. That's a whole lotta fake boobies!! (Read in an Adam Sandler, from *The Wedding Singer*, voice.)

We have frequently been asked: Can you breast-feed after a boob job? Despite the large number of these surgeries, few medical studies have researched this issue. The only available studies clearly indicate a greater incidence of insufficient lactation among augmented women compared with nonaugmented women. The type of surgical approach is especially important in determining whether breast-feeding may be a problem. In most breast augmentations, one of three types of incisions is made: an incision underneath the breast, an incision around the lower edge of the nipple (areola), or an incision within the armpit. The periareolar approach is most significantly associated with lactation insufficiency. Surgical technique is also key, as the ability to breast-feed may be impaired when too many milk ducts are severed.

3:50 p.m.

Gberg: Oh, I forgot to tell you, I spoke to Penny yesterday and warned her that now she is vulnerable to our IM insults in the book.

Leyner: Penny—she doesn't deserve our bilious insults like Carrie does.

Gberg: She said her husband wondered if any diseases could swim upstream while peeing in a public urinal.

Leyner: WHAT?

Gberg: Like salmon going to lay their eggs?

Gberg: Did I say public urinal? Is there another kind?

Leyner: Of course ... private urinals.

Gberg: You need a membership card.

Leyner: Isn't that a Tina Turner song? "Private Urinal"?

Gberg: Yes, please serenade me!

Leyner: *Saving Private Urinal* ... Spielberg's attempt at depicting the homoerotic splendors of the Port Authority men's room ...

Leyner: Ahead of its time ...

Gberg: A classic.

Gberg: I also wondered why they called those things urinal cakes.

3:55 p.m.

Gberg: Not much like dessert.

Leyner: I thought they were like those little British tea sandwiches.

Gberg: Cucumber sandwiches and urinal cakes. Doesn't get classier than that.

Gberg: That's klassy with a k.

Leyner: That's what I'm talkin' about!!!! Lord Nelson would be proud of YOU right now. Grog, a urinal cake, and a cat-o'-nine-tails ... You got an afternoon's delight right there, sailor.

Gberg: Skyrockets in flight.

Leyner: Remember that scene in that Will Ferrell *Anchorman* movie where they sing that in the office?

Gberg: Yes. I still love when he's so thirsty and drinks the milk.

Gberg: Milk was a bad choice!

Leyner: It's one of those philosophical conundrums akin to the unheard tree falling in the woods.

Leyner: Do you ever drink milk?

Gberg: Only when I want a lot of mucus!

Leyner: I want a lot of mucus!!!

4:00 p.m.

Leyner: I'm very acquisitive.

Gberg: Actually, that's not true. We are going to answer that question in the book.

Leyner: I want a lot of money and A LOT OF MUCUS.

Leyner: Milk doesn't give me mucus ... if you need definitive empirical data on the subject.

Leyner: Milk gives me a great sense of blithe optimism.

Leyner: Carrie gives me a lot of mucus.

Leyner: Every time I hear the name "Carrie" and the phrase "Where is the manuscript?" I hawk up spit.

Gberg: I think our next project together should be a musical.

4:05 p.m.

Leyner: You know that French chick who fed her face to her own dog and then got a transplant.

If ever there was an obvious case of
Münchausen's syndrome, that was it.

Leyner: I'm making myself laugh a lot here, by
the way.

Gberg: Good, I'm glad you are entertaining yourself.

Gberg: Hey, I am working on the pregnancy chapter. Did you ever read that breast-feeding and
fake boobs article?

Leyner: No, not yet ... I'm sticking to my assigned
purviews.

Leyner: Tell me about it ...

Gberg: I was hoping you were going to add some
great humor but thanks for nothing.

4:10 p.m.

Leyner: I can read it right now, if you want.

Leyner: Give me ten minutes.

Gberg: No, do your sections. I don't want to dis-
tract a master at work.

Leyner: And we'll discuss ... like Oprah's Book
Club.

Leyner: Do you think ...

Leyner: Do you think that a mother who's had
breast augmentation has an ethical obligation
to tell her pubescent daughter ... so that the
daughter can factor that into her expectation
for how big her breasts might grow to be?

4:15 p.m.

Leyner: You didn't answer my question about the mom with the boob job and the pubescent daughter.

Leyner: Plastic surgery makes it impossible for children to extrapolate what they're going to look like.

Gberg: Did you hear the one about the priest, the rabbi, the mom with the boob job, and the pre-pubescent daughter?

Gberg: Doesn't make sense to extrapolate any-way. Genetics is some crazy stuff.

Leyner: You can't just look at your own parents ... you might have the boobs of your grandma ... is that what you're saying?

Gberg: Ever see pictures of some models with their mothers and the mother looks like a car-nival freak who just escaped from a trailer park?

Gberg: Oh man, those steam pipes are banging again at my house. They are driving me crazy.

Leyner: You're getting me all hot and bothered ... I was picturing myself in a room at the Ritz Carleton in San Juan with a model and her carnival-freak mother ...

Leyner: I'm slathering that Spanish caramel gook all over the trailer-park mom.

Gberg: We should go away somewhere to work on this beast of a book and put it to rest.

Leyner: What's that stuff called ...? Dulce something or other.

Gberg: Dulce de leche.

4:20 p.m.

Gberg: Do you know how they make it?

Leyner: Yes ... dulce de leche is excellent slathered on the pale hairless bodies of carnival freaks.

Leyner: How do they make it?

Gberg: You just take an unopened can of condensed milk and stick it in a pot of water for an hour.

Leyner: And ...

Gberg: Tastes delicious with anything.

Leyner: Ummmmm ...

Leyner: What a great idea ... dulce de leche and grilled baby octopus ...

Gberg: We could write a cookbook.

Leyner: You could add it to short ribs or a porkbelly sandwich.

4:25 p.m.

Leyner: Or swordfish with papaya salsa ... OR ...

Leyner: Do you know the story about the man who was sitting on a toilet in the Port Authority men's room—and a swordfish who'd gotten lost somehow and had wandered from the Atlantic into the Hudson River and somehow errantly swam into the NYC sewer system—swam up the toilet and buried its sword into the anus hole of the hapless defecating man ... remember that?

Gberg: You are a troubled young man.

4:30 p.m.

Leyner: I'm somnambulant and pure energy and my business parts are as sweet as dulce de leche.

Leyner: I'm an INCUBUS.

Gberg: What is an incubus?

Leyner: A spirit that has sexual intercourse with women while they are sleeping.

Gberg: Well, that you are.

Leyner: Thank you.

Gberg: All right, I have to get back to answering some of these darn questions.

Leyner: OK. It was nice chatting with you. You are charming and erudite.

Gberg: You are erudite and charming.

Leyner: You know what the female version of an incubus is?

Gberg: A succubus.

Leyner: Bingo.

Leyner: Bye. Have a nice life.

Leyner: I mean it. I'm so outta here.

Can you breast-feed with a nipple piercing?

We have actually been asked if nipple piercing will result in a lawn-sprinkler effect when you lactate. There is no evidence to suggest that a woman's pierced nipples will have any effect on her ability to breast-feed. That is, if there haven't been any complications resulting from the procedure. Infection and scarring are frequent complications after nipple piercing.

It is hard to imagine a pierced mother not removing the nipple ring prior to breast-feeding, but alas, some insist on keeping themselves festooned despite recommendations to the contrary. In these cases, breast-feeding difficulties include poor latch, gagging, and milk leaking from the baby's mouth. But if you insist on wearing your jewelry, make sure that it is firmly attached, since you definitely don't want the baby to swallow it and choke!

Do your feet really grow when you are pregnant?

There is a whole lot of growing going on in pregnancy. Most growth is done by the little baby inside, but some of the growth is passed on to Mom. The belly and the boobs are the most obvious, but the extra weight caused in pregnancy also increases pressure on a pregnant woman's feet.

Hormonal changes are also occurring that relax the ligaments in the body to prepare for delivery. The specifics of these hormonal changes are not fully understood, but one hormone, relaxin, is thought to contribute to the loosening of ligaments in the pelvis and elsewhere.

The work of gravity and relaxin cause the arch of the foot to lose its strength and the tissue on the bottom of the foot, the plantar fascia, to stretch. All of this makes the foot grow wider and flatter during pregnancy. The feet can even grow by more than one shoe size.

After delivery, the body begins to return to normal and many of these changes reverse themselves. If the changes were extreme during pregnancy and the ligaments were significantly stretched, the increased shoe size could be permanent.

Why did rabbits die in old pregnancy tests?

Hopefully, most of you have forgotten the 1978 film *Rabbit Test*, directed by Joan Rivers, starring Billy Crystal as the world's first pregnant man. If you haven't heard of it, know this, it should have died like the rabbits in the early pregnancy tests.

The original pregnancy test really was a "rabbit

test" and the rabbit always died. In the 1920s, scientists discovered a hormone known as human chorionic gonadotropin (hCG) that was produced early in pregnancy. It was also discovered that when injected into certain animals, the hCG would cause changes in animal ovaries. The first test, discovered by Selmar Aschheim and Bernhard Zondek, was performed on mice. In 1931, Maurice H. Friedman refined the test by using rabbits, and the rabbit or Friedman test was born. Human urine was injected into a rabbit and forty-eight hours later, the rabbit was killed and its ovaries were examined to determine if the person was pregnant or not.

Modern pregnancy tests are still based on measuring the amount of hCG present in urine or blood, without the use of a rabbit. The first home pregnancy tests were approved in 1976. Raucous celebrations were held in many rabbit families.

Why do you get hairier when you are pregnant?

Many women notice that the hair on their head is thicker during pregnancy. They also may notice some new growth on their chin, upper lip, cheeks, breasts, belly, arms, legs, and back. Don't worry, this growth is often subtle, and you won't end up looking like a Wookie.

Pregnancy-induced hair growth usually develops during the first trimester. Just like most pregnancy

changes, it is caused by a change in hormones. This
growth usually abates six months after delivery. Some
women may notice increased shedding of hair during
this period. This is simply your body adjusting as hormone levels return to normal.

Do pregnant women really glow?

If a pregnant woman asks her husband, "Am I glow-
ing?" there is only one answer: "Yes, dear."

Don't worry about lying; the pregnancy glow actually exists and has a biological basis. In pregnancy,
blood volume increases by almost 50 percent. This
increased blood volume causes the cheeks of women
to take on a reddish blush. Pregnancy hormones also
cause increased secretions from the oil glands, and
this leaves the face nice and shiny. The end result ... a
beautiful glow.

But not all of pregnancy's dermatological changes
are pleasant. We already mentioned that you can get
hairier. You also may develop spider veins in your legs
from the increased blood flow and hormones.

Skin over the stretching abdomen can become
very itchy, and you also may be unlucky enough to
develop PUPP or pruritic urticarial papules and
plaques of pregnancy. This is a fancy term for itchy
bumps that develop in the second half of pregnancy
on the abdomen, thighs, butt, and legs of about 1
percent of pregnant women.

Why do your nipples turn brown in pregnancy?

If you have dark skin, you may have brown nipples before pregnancy, but many pregnant women of all complexions notice that their nipples have become somewhat darker.

As we keep mentioning, pregnancy causes changes in hormone levels, duh! In this case, an increase in estrogen levels and melanocyte-stimulating-hormone (MSH) levels causes the changes. MSH acts on melanocytes. These are cells within the skin that determine the degree of pigmentation. The face and the belly are two areas where darkening of the skin can be most noticeable.

Some pregnant women experience the "mask of pregnancy" or chloasma, an array of brownish or yellowish patches on the facial skin, unevenly distributed on the forehead, temples, and middle of the face. This is more common in women with dark hair and pale skin. Chloasma cannot be prevented, but you can minimize the intensity of these darkened areas by limiting your exposure to sunlight. These marks will usually fade completely after delivery.

Then there is the dark line on the belly, the linea negra. In many women, there is a normal faint (barely visible) white line, the linea alba, running from the navel to the center of their pubic bone. During pregnancy in the second trimester, extra pigment in the skin causes a darkening of this line. The linea nigra is

darker in darker-skinned women and fades after
delivery too.

What causes severe leg cramps at night during pregnancy?

Has your pregnant wife begged you to rub her legs?
Have you noticed that occasionally she shakes her leg
like a dog having its belly rubbed?

Here is another problem that women experience
in pregnancy, the presence of leg cramps. Some
women also can get an uncomfortable, jittery sensation running in both legs known as restless leg syndrome. These conditions are intermittent, but they
can be very disturbing, particularly at night.

Leg cramps have always been a difficult condition
for doctors to treat. Leg cramps affect almost half of
all pregnant women, but the cause of leg cramps during pregnancy is not fully understood. Leg cramps are
more common in the second and third trimesters of
pregnancy and happen most often at night. Cramps
may be the result of the extra weight carried during
this time and the pressure that it places on the legs.
Changes in circulation also can affect the legs. Some
older theories have been that deficiencies in salt,
magnesium, or calcium caused these cramps, but no
study has shown any connection to calcium. Sodium
supplementation might decrease the number of leg
cramps in pregnancy, but the effect is very small. The

benefit for magnesium is stronger. Magnesium supplementation (magnesium lactate or citrate) might help and low doses shouldn't be harmful. Be sure, however, to ask your doctor before taking any supplements.

Other simple tips for leg cramps include:

- Stay well hydrated.
- Stretch and massage your calf muscles.
- Exercise.
- Blame your husband for getting you into this mess!

Is it true that babies can be born with teeth?

Sounds like a scene from a horror film. A baby is delivered and opens its mouth to reveal a full set of chompers. Then the little devil begins to chew his way through the delivery-room staff ...

It ain't gonna happen! But scary as it sounds, babies *can* be born with teeth. They are called natal teeth and these teeth are present at the time of birth. Neonatal teeth erupt within thirty days of delivery.

Natal teeth generally develop on the lower gum and there are usually only two or three of them. They don't have strong roots and are often loose. Natal teeth are uncommon, and found in only one in every 2,000 to 6,000 births. Natal teeth may cause irritation and trauma to the infant's tongue while he or she is nursing. They also may be uncomfortable for a nursing mother. (No kidding!)

If the natal teeth are loose, they should be removed shortly after birth while the newborn infant is still in the hospital. A loose natal tooth could be swallowed and the child could be at risk for aspiration.

Should pregnant women avoid cats and kitty litter?

This is all about toxoplasmosis, an infection caused by a parasite called *Toxoplasma gondii*. Cat feces and kitty litter are a major source of toxoplasmosis since cats are a natural host for this parasite that reproduces in their intestines. Toxoplasmosis can also be found in raw or undercooked meat or in contaminated soil. The Centers for Disease Control (CDC) estimate that only about 15 percent of women of childbearing age are immune to toxoplasmosis. The infection caused by the parasite is minor in healthy individuals, but the risk lies in the fact that this infection could be passed on to your baby.

An estimated 400 to 4,000 cases of congenital toxoplasmosis occur in the United States each year. Congenital toxoplasmosis can cause miscarriage, stillbirth, or death shortly after birth. Congenital toxoplasmosis can also affect your baby's brain, causing mental retardation, seizures, blindness, and death.

Don't fear: most cases of congenital toxoplasmosis can be prevented by educating women of childbearing age and pregnant women to avoid eating raw or undercooked meat, and wear gloves while gardening and, if possible, have someone else change the kitty litter. (If you're pregnant and you have to clean the cat's commode, try to wear gloves and be sure to wash carefully.)

Can squirting breast milk in a baby's eye help a clogged tear duct?

This question came from Billy's sister, who gained nationwide notoriety during an embarrassing moment on *The Today Show*, when the host Matt Lauer revealed that she referred to her brother as "Dummy Doctor." So how does she expect Dummy Doctor to be able to answer obscure questions like this one? She should know that there is no class in medical school on the ocular applications of breast milk.

We *were* able to find some references to the therapeutic uses of breast milk. Human breast milk contains various antimicrobial compounds. Some of these compounds have been shown to fight off bacteria such as *Escherichia coli*, *Salmonella enteritidis*, and *Staphylococcus epidermidis*.

If your baby has a clogged tear duct, the first step

is to see your pediatrician. The doctor will probably teach you to gently wipe the yellow discharge out of your baby's eyes and to massage the tear ducts. You also can apply breast milk if you are breastfeeding. All you need to do is express a couple drops of your milk onto the tip of a clean finger and gently place them in the corner of the draining eye.

Can sleeping on your back hurt the baby?

When a pregnant woman arrives at the hospital in labor, we tell her to lie on her left side rather than lying flat on her back. The rationale behind this is that on your back, the baby can cause compression of the vena cava, a major blood vessel that passes under the uterus. During labor, a contraction itself can reduce blood flow to the baby and that compression on this vessel can exacerbate this decrease in blood flow.

A healthy baby can tolerate this without any difficulty, especially if you are not in labor. So don't worry if you sleep on your back. Get rest while you still have a chance.

Why shouldn't pregnant women dye their hair?

There are several studies that look at the relationship between maternal hair dyes and childhood diseases, including childhood brain tumors. Don't expect to find any information that praises the health benefits of hair dyeing, but you won't find any evidence that it is particularly dangerous either.

Even though there are no studies linking hair dyes to any prenatal toxicity, many conservative doctors tell their patients to pass on going platinum until after the baby is born. The truth is that it is probably fine to get some highlights and an occasional color rinse, but you probably shouldn't soak your head in a vat of dye nightly—plus, your hair would fall out.

Will playing music to your baby make it calmer, smarter, and healthier?

We had to send Leyner—that polyglot punk—to the Bulgarian literature on this one. In a 2004 edition of *Akusherstvo i Ginekologiia*, he came across an article about the "Effect of Music on Fetal Behavior." This study found that music stimulation did cause changes in fetal heart rate and body movement. Other studies have tried to evaluate whether exposure to music in utero could lead to fetal learning and they found similar responses.

Theoretically, exposure to music could lead to learning, but there isn't any science to support this. Some call the possible connection the "Mozart Effect," but there isn't any proof that listening to *The Magic Flute* will produce a prodigy.

If you believe in the Mozart Effect, you can probably wait until about week twenty-four, because that is when the fetus begins to recognize sounds.

Are summer pregnancies more likely to result in twins?

There are several studies that have sought to determine a relationship between twin birth rate and the season of birth. Other studies have examined the effects of temperature on human fertility. When you look carefully at all of these studies, there is a slight but statistically significant tendency for conceptions that occur in summer to result in twins.

Some think that this is a result of sunlight stimulating the hormone FSH in women, which in turn increases the likelihood of a multiple birth.

Is it true that all babies are born with blue eyes?

Blue eyes,
Baby's got blue eyes.
—Elton John

Need we say more? Well, maybe we should at least explain a little. Eye color is determined by the amount of a single pigment called melanin that is present in the iris of the eye. Melanin is a dark-brown pigment. If a lot of melanin is present, the eye will appear brown or even black. If very little melanin is present, the iris will appear blue. Less melanin produces green, gray, or light-brown eyes.

In general, Caucasian babies are born with blue eyes because melanin hasn't been deposited in the irises of their eyes yet. African, Asian, Hispanic, and Native American babies, on the other hand, are often born with brown or black eyes. Melanin production generally increases during the first few months of a baby's life, after which eye color changes and the color is stable by about six months of age.

Is it true that some people eat the placenta?

The closest thing that we found when looking for documentation of human placentophagia was that certain mammals do eat the placenta. Oh, and Billy's friend Gail likes polenta. But that really doesn't have much to do with the answer.

The Internet has many references to eating the placenta and recipes abound. It is unclear whether this is actually done. Many ancient cultures revered the placenta. The Navajo felt that the placenta was sacred but poisonous. The Shilluk, a Sudanese people on the West Nile, apparently practiced a symbolic ingestion of the afterbirth. They buried the placenta at the roots of a fruit tree, and the following season ritualistically ate the fruit and drank tea made from the fruit. Human placenta has also been an ingredient in some traditional Chinese medicines.

Does having a lot of heartburn mean the baby has a full head of hair?

Heartburn or acid reflux is extremely common when pregnant. During pregnancy, the placenta produces the hormone progesterone, which serves to relax the smooth muscles of the uterus. Progesterone also relaxes the smooth muscle in the sphincter between the esophagus and the stomach. This allows stomach acids to sneak up the esophagus, causing heartburn. Progesterone also slows down the wave-like contractions of the stomach, making digestion sluggish. It doesn't help that you have a large baby inside who is pushing on your stomach.

Knowing all this, if heartburn caused babies to grow hair, most newborns would look like little chimps. This one is definitely a myth.

Does eating fish make the baby smarter?

This one gets rather complicated.

Recently, there have been many warnings for pregnant women to avoid certain kinds of fish in order to prevent mercury poisoning. Shark, swordfish, king mackerel, and golden or white snapper are to be avoided because they contain high levels of potentially brain-damaging mercury. It is generally recommended that pregnant women have only two servings of fish (ones that are low in mercury) a week, but these warnings may lead women to eat even less.

On the other hand, there is evidence that the fatty acids in fish may also help prenatal brains develop. This is where the problems really start. Eat too much fish and you risk potential problems with mercury poisoning. Eat too little and you might deprive the developing brain of fatty acids that may make your baby smarter.

Docosahexaenoic acid (DHA), an omega-3 long-chain polyunsaturated fatty acid, is the main fatty acid that is found in fish and that is needed for brain development. Some nutritionists recommend that pregnant women get their DHA through algae-derived supplements. Omega-3-fortified eggs are another good source of DHA.

Chapter 6

Eyes, Ears, Mouth, and Nose

I t was another day at the therapeutic offices of Leyner and Dr. Billy. Leyner was especially happy— he was listening to his new iPod and had just down-loaded an obscure but remarkable hip-hop version of Verdi's *Rigoletto*. Our next clients were a family we'd never encountered before. This was their first session. And it was quite a revelation to see them gathered in the waiting room—father, mother, and five children of vary-ing ages from five to fifteen. The extraordinary thing was how they were dressed. They were each arrayed in matching outfits—shiny orange polyester shirts, with lemon-yellow vests, and sky-blue slacks. Each wore an individually colored kerchief knotted around his or her neck.

Wendy shepherded the colorfully attired flock into the office.

The mother spoke first, in an angelic voice. "Is he going to listen to his headphones the whole session?"

I elbowed Leyner and he responded far too loudly, "Dude, I'm listening to 'Questa o Quella.' Can you wait a minute?"

I shrugged and apologized to the family. "He's just getting in the mood for the session. So what brings you here today?"

The mother reached inside her bra and withdrew a pitch pipe and blew a clear, dulcet note. She turned to her family and they began to sing a chorale rendition of Kelly Clarkson's *American Idol*-winning ballad, "A Moment Like This."

The music was beautiful and ethereal, but occasionally a harsh discordant sound would emerge from among the younger children. The mother silenced them one by one until only a sheepish six-year-old boy was singing, shifting his weight uneasily from foot to foot, his head bowed. He stopped, knowing that he was the culprit responsible for the squeaky sound that ruined an otherwise perfect performance.

The family remained mute, but Leyner ripped off his headphones and added, "Man, what was that horrible sound?!"

The father silenced him with a glare. "This is why we are here!"

I gently quizzed the family to learn more about their difficulties. It turned out that little Richard was a wonderful brother and son. He excelled in all his academic pursuits and was an all-star forward in his junior soccer league. Unfortunately, he couldn't carry a tune to save his life, which in this family was an unforgivable sin.

I discovered that since infancy, Richard had experienced terrible trouble with music. The worried family had consulted expert after expert, and even traveled to Vienna to consult the world's leading specialist in congenital amusia, Dr. Amanda von Binkenstein. As various family members recounted the ignominy of growing up with their hapless atonal sibling, poor little Richard slumped further and further into his chair, his face reddening with embarrassment.

I couldn't in good conscience allow the humiliation of this boy to continue much longer without intervening. I turned to Leyner. "Do me a favor, sing for this nice family."

Leyner jumped out of his seat. "Really? Can I put on one of those outfits?" Leyner saw my disapproval, but added anyway, "Can I at least get a pitch pipe?"

He then began to sing one of the most god-awful versions of "Lady Marmalade" that you could ever imagine. The whole family was wincing in pain except for little Richard. The more hopelessly off-key Leyner got, the happier it seemed to make the boy, who couldn't take his eyes off my shamelessly caterwauling partner.

When Leyner finally finished, little Richard stood and applauded. In a devilish voice, he said, "You're my hero. You suck even worse than I do."

The ashamed mother grabbed her son and scolded him. "Richard, apologize to that nice man. Not everyone is a star at everything. We each have our special innate talents."

I looked into her eyes and she caught herself.

"Hmmm," sang the entire family in unison, nodding their heads in assent with their mother's therapeutic revelation. They embraced little Richard.

Leyner tried to interrupt. "I was just warming up. Can I sing another number?"

The father turned to Leyner and responded, "Don't quit your day job," as the family strolled away.

I was left to console a bitterly wounded Leyner, who was left muttering, "What the hell do they know about music!"

Are some people really tone deaf?

All you have to do is listen to Billy and his wife sing in the car and you will know that the answer is yes.

Tone deafness is the inability to recognize musical tones or reproduce them. It is also called amusia or dysmelodia. This can occur after a traumatic brain injury, but it can also be present from birth. Congenital amusia is the most common term used for tone deafness that is present from birth.

If you want to read about the first reported case of tone deafness, just go to the 1878 journal *Mind* and read Grant-Allen's article "Note-Deafness." The article describes the case of a thirty-year-old man who took music lessons as a child, but was completely unable to carry a tune or recognize familiar melodies.

Congenital amusia is similar to a learning disability. Patients do not have any brain injury, hearing loss, or other cognitive deficit.

The other end of the spectrum is perfect pitch or absolute pitch, the ability to recognize a pitch without any external reference. Perfect pitch is thought to involve both genetic and environmental factors.

Why do you sneeze when you stare at the sun?

This is definitely one of those things that you don't learn in medical school, and we were amazed when we found out that there was a real answer to this question.

Yes, some people do sneeze when they look at the sun. This is due to something called the photic sneeze reflex. It is also known as autosomal dominant compelling helio-ophthalmic outburst or ACHOO, solar sneezing, and photosternutatory reflex. The photic sneeze reflex usually causes more than one sneeze. A study of six Spanish families showed that sneezes occur with a frequency of two to three sneezes per sneezing episode, with about three seconds between each sneeze. The photic sneeze reflex occurs in approximately 10 to 25 percent of the population, but even sun-sneezers don't do it all the time.

This reflex is not completely understood, but it is thought to occur due to an accidental crossing of nerve signals in the fifth cranial nerve nucleus. This reflex trait is genetic and is passed on in an autosomal dominant manner. That means that if one of your parents is a sun-sneezer, you have a 50 percent chance of being a sun-sneezer too.

If you read the journal *Military Medicine*, you might also know that the photic sneeze reflex is also considered a risk factor to combat pilots.

Does your heart stop when you sneeze?

When you sneeze, it changes the pressure inside your chest (intrathoracic pressure) and this affects blood flow to the heart. This alteration in blood flow can temporarily affect the beating of the heart, but it most definitely will not stop.

By the way, the medical term for a sneeze is sternutation. Throw that one around and even some doctors won't know what you are talking about.

What are the lines going down from the nose to the lip?

Billy's mother worked as a genetic counselor at a center for craniofacial disorders. It was a common family event for Mama Goldberg to comment on the philtrum of someone whom she passed on the street. Yes, that vertical groove in the upper lip is called the philtrum. It comes from the Greek word *philtron*, which means love charm.

The philtrum is formed in embryonic development when the medial nasal prominences fuse, between the sixth and seventh week. The philtrum still needs more refining to achieve its ultimate form, usually by week fourteen.

Children with fetal alcohol syndrome are often described as having a flat philtrum. Short philtrums and long philtrums are seen in various genetic diseases. If you need more details, just call Billy's mom, she would love to talk about them.

What causes ringing in the ears?

Doctors always prefer an esoteric word to describe a simple condition. So they call ringing in the ears tinnitus.

Tinnitus is very common, with about 36 million sufferers in the United States. There are many different things that cause a ringing in the ears. Some of these are extremely common and most are not very serious, while other causes can be very dangerous. Causes include age-related hearing loss (presbycusis), trauma, medications (aspirin, antibiotics), changes in ear bones, atherosclerosis, high blood pressure, head and neck tumors, TMJ, Ménière's disease, ear infection, thyroid disease, increased blood flow, and wax buildup.

Most commonly, tinnitus develops when there is some damage to the hearing apparatus, or the hair cells inside the ears. These are tiny little protrusions that cover the cochlea inside the inner ear. When noises are perceived, these tiny hair cells send electrical signals to the brain that are turned into sound. Some experts think that tinnitus may originate in the brain rather than in the ear.

Famous tinnitus sufferers:

- Beethoven.
- Michelangelo.
- Charles Darwin.
- William Shatner (Captain James T. Kirk).

Is eye color genetic?

Did you fall asleep in the back of biology class or what? Don't you remember Gregor Mendel, the Austrian monk and his pea plants? Mendel was considered to be the Father of Genetics, and if you were listening in high school instead of shooting spitballs, you might remember his round and wrinkled pea pods and the simple laws of inheritance. Unfortunately, these simple laws don't apply to eye color.

The common assumption that is taught in schools is that brown eye color is always dominant to blue, and that two blue-eyed parents will always produce a blue-eyed child. This is not always true. Two blue-eyed parents can produce children with brown eyes. This happens because eye color is determined by many genes (polygenic) rather than by one.

Eye color is determined by the amount of a pigment called melanin that is in the iris of the eye. Brown eyes have a lot of pigment, and blue eyes have very little. The eye-color genes control enzymes that direct the amount of melanin in the iris.

Although eye color is assumed to remain constant over the course of your entire life, this too can change. Eyes can change color as an individual ages or as the result of some diseases. Eye color can also change from trauma, and sometimes there are drug-induced changes that can occur from the treatment of glaucoma.

Why do your eyes water when you pooh?

Okay, well, maybe it doesn't happen to everyone when they pooh, but someone who will remain nameless is known to get teary during a good move-ment. (Okay, it's Dr. Billy.) For the rest of you, yawning may make your eyes water and the reason is prob-ably the same.

The theory is that during a yawn or a good pooh, you scrunch up the muscles of the face. The contrac-tion of these muscles can force the tear ducts and glands to be compressed and that forces out tears.

There are three main types of tears: basal tears (lubricate the eye), reflex tears (think onions), and emotional tears. We suggest a fourth category: pooh tears.

Why do some people have two different-color eyes?

I (Dr. Billy) have a special attachment to this question. I have had two dear friends who both had two different-color eyes. Ramsey, I am sorry that I am putting you in the same group with Winnie, the Old English sheep dog that we had growing up, but he was special too.

Heterochromia iridium is the fancy medical name for two different-color eyes in the same person. This is relatively rare in humans, but can be seen frequently in some animals, such as Siamese cats and Australian shepherds. Heterochromia can be the result of an inherited trait, a medical syndrome, or a physical accident. It is thought to result from a change in one of the genes that controls eye color.

A variation on this condition is heterochromia iridis, where different parts of a single eye vary in color. This occurs when one part of the iris has a different amount of pigment (melanin) due to injury, drugs, disease, or a simple birthmark.

Nowadays, all you need is a fancy set of contact lenses and you can have instant heterochromia—just like Marilyn Manson.

Are your eyeballs the size at birth that they will be your whole life?

Babies seem to have enormous eyes so it is not surprising that people ask this question. Newborn eyes are about 18 millimeters in diameter. Depending on the source, this is anywhere from two-thirds to three-quarters of the fully grown adult size. So, no, they are not the adult size at birth.

Most eye growth does occur in the first year of life, however, and by the time you are three, your eye growth is nearly complete.

Do iPods cause hearing loss?

Hearing experts worry that the increasing popularity of MP3 players may lead to widespread hearing loss. The concern is that with increased sound quality, people are listening to music louder and longer.

Music and loud noise have been known to cause hearing loss for centuries. Noise exposure causes hearing loss by damaging the hair cells in the cochlea of the inner ear. The hair cells transmit sound information to your brain. Hair cells can recover from temporary damage, but loud and frequent noise can permanently damage them. A good way to understand the temporary damage is to compare it with walking on grass. If you walk on a lawn occasionally, you won't damage it because the grass has a chance to recover. If you trample the grass constantly, it loses its ability to bounce back and becomes permanently damaged. Damage to the hair cells in the ear happens the same way.

The decibel (dB) is the unit used to measure sound levels. The cutoff for acceptable risk for workplace noise is 85 dB. The level of negligible risk is considered to be 75 dB or below. Many studies have looked at personal stereos and, in general, listening levels tend to be below the 85 dB risk cutoff. A study in the April 2005 *International Journal of Audiology* looked at noise-exposure levels from personal-stereo use and determined that the average continuous noise-exposure level was 79.8 dB, with a statistically significant difference between males and females, of 80.6 dB and 75.3 dB respectively. Basically, most people stay within a safe range, but it is important to watch the volume, because some personal music players reportedly can produce levels as high as 120 dB.

Here are some other estimates of noise levels:

30 dB	whisper
60 dB	normal conversation
80 dB	ringing telephone
90 dB	hair dryer/power lawnmower
93 dB	belt sander
96 dB	tractor
98 dB	hand drill

108 dB	continuous miner
110 dB	chain saw
114 dB	hammer drill
120 dB	ambulance siren
140 dB	jet engine at takeoff
165 dB	12-gauge shotgun
180 dB	rocket launch
194 dB	loudest tone possible

So … the bottom line is that if you are driving an ambulance to the shooting range, you should use ear protection. As for the iPod, we love everything that Apple makes so we hope that they aren't dangerous. We suggest that you keep the volume low, but even if they find out that iPods cause hearing loss, imagine the cool hearing aids that Steve Jobs will create.

4:35 p.m.

Gberg: Give me a call on the home phone so we can talk about the cover.

Leyner: Maybe.

Leyner: See you in the future.

Leyner: And remember one thing:

Leyner: I didn't ask to be born.

Gberg: Don't leave me this way.

Leyner: OK … I love you … I'll never forget the time in Venice when you sang "Afternoon Delight" to me in the gondola right after my

bilateral inguinal hernia repair ... I'll never forget your kindness that summer ...

Leyner: OK? Is that better?

Gberg: Who sang "Afternoon Delight"?

Leyner: Trini Lopez and Garth Brooks?

Gberg: I just cheated and went on to iTunes.

Gberg: They have a Will Ferrell version from
Anchorman.

Leyner: I'd say buy it ... but I know you're too
cheap.

Gberg: You have hurt my feelings once again.

What are those dust particles you sometimes see floating in front of your eyes?

In our last book, we called one of Billy's smartest
friends for the composition of eye bogeys. This
Proust-reading, NPR-listening, Ivy League-educated
retina surgeon came up empty, but we decided to
give him another chance. This time, not only did we
get an answer, but we also got a quote from ol'
Marcel Proust:

... we feel a veritable fever of yearning for the fallen leaves
that can go so far as to keep us awake at night. Into my
closed room they had been drifting already for a month,
summoned there by my desire to see them, slipping

between my thoughts and the object, whatever it might be, upon which I was trying to concentrate them, whirling in front of me like those brown spots that sometimes, whatever we may be looking at, will seem to be dancing or swimming before our eyes.

—Remembrance of Things Past: Swann's Way,
p. 456., trans. C. K. Scott Moncrieff
and Terence Kilmartin, Random House

These floating spots are very common and arise because our eyes are filled with a clear gel, called vitreous humor, which, as time goes by, can partially liquefy to form small condensations, opacities, and debris. These opacities float through the vitreous as the eye moves, casting shadows on the retina (the light-sensing neural tissue lining the back of the eye). We perceive these shadows as "floaters." In medical-speak, they are called vitreous floaters or migratory scotomata. They resemble cobwebs or gnats or even tiny paisleys that slowly drift through the field of vision.

Most of the time floaters are benign, but in rare cases they can signal a serious problem such as a retinal tear or detachment. If you are concerned and are in San Francisco, look up Billy's friend, and you can get a consultation and perhaps a lecture on French literature.

1:25 p.m.

Gberg: Leyner. Are you out there?

Gberg: Hello.

Gberg: Won't you light my candle?

Leyner: What? You buttwad ...

1:30 p.m.

Gberg: Just got your TV question.

Leyner: I'm getting great at this!! I've finally found my true métier.

Leyner: Should we put it in puberty?

Gberg: I think it is great. What about sitting too close and being bad for the eyes?

Leyner: Good separate question. Let's keep that one in our bag of tricks ... and if we need more later, we'll take that one on too.

Leyner: How about this? My mom asked me last night ...

Gberg: Yes.

Leyner: Why do we see shapes and patterns and colors when we close our eyes?

Leyner: Interesting, boring??

Leyner: Can't decide.

Leyner: Let's put that aside too, yes?

Gberg: We have a question about floaters. That might satisfy Mama's curiosity.

Leyner: I love that TV one, though.

Leyner: OK, let's stick with the floaters.

Gberg: Yeah, baby. We are getting there.

Leyner: I think we're going to be very proud of
this book.

Leyner: I really think it's better.

Gberg: We got another bad Amazon review criti-
cizing the IMs.

Leyner: I'm going to the gym ... I'll call you on the
way and we'll talk about the IMs ...

Gberg: Make that 2.

1:35 p.m.

Leyner: 2 about the IMs?

Gberg: "Disappointing application of an excellent
premise" and "Boring and uncouth."

Gberg: I think we should dedicate the book to
these armchair critics.

1:40 p.m.

Gberg: Did I lose you?

Leyner: I'm back.

Leyner: Stop reading all that shit. THAT will certainly rot your brain.

Leyner: Are you reassessing the IMing ... ? Let's
talk about it.

Leyner: I'll call you in a few minutes ... Are you
going to sleep soon?

1:45 p.m.

Gberg: Call my cell. I am going over to Bar Pitti.

Gberg: Drown my sorrow in rigatoni and red
wine.

> **Leyner:** OK ... I'll call your cell. Fuck those idiots
> at Amazon ... Why do you read that garbage?
> Bye.

When water is stuck in your ears, where is it? How do you get it out?

People have this strange idea that if water gets in your ear, it will somehow find its way to the inside of your skull. The truth is that if your eardrum is intact, the water will remain in your outer ear canal. But, besides being uncomfortable, this water creates an environment where infections can develop.

Swimmer's ear or otitis externa is an infection of the lining of the external ear canal that begins when water gets stuck in the outer ear. This is different from a regular or middle ear infection, which is an infection behind the eardrum. There also is a condition called surfer's ear or exostosis of the external auditory canal. Surfer's ear is caused by repeated exposure to cold water and wind. This cooling of the ear canal causes bone growth that eventually blocks the ear canal.

If your ear is kept dry, it is unlikely to become infected. You can opt for earplugs or rely on the old jump-up-and-down-on-one-leg-and-bang-the-side-of-your-head-with-your-hand-with-your-bad-ear-toward-the-floor trick. Cotton buds should be avoided because they can push material deep into the canal or scratch the skin, making infection more likely.

Other options include ear-drying drops to evaporate excess water or a hair dryer to dry them out. There even are rechargeable ear dryers that are specially designed for this purpose.

Does thumb-sucking cause buckteeth?

Thumb-sucking is a normal behavior. Well, sucking your own thumb is normal. If you are sucking someone else's, that's a little weird!

Thumb-sucking only becomes a problem if it continues for too long. It can begin during the fetal period, but should be curtailed by the time that permanent teeth come in. Permanent teeth begin to sprout around age six. If thumb-sucking continues past this age, your child can develop an overbite or buckteeth.

There are other problems that come along with late thumb-sucking. An article in 1993 in the journal *Pediatrics* looked at the "influence of thumb-sucking on peer social acceptance in first-grade children." They found that thumb-sucking children were judged as less intelligent, happy, attractive, likable, and fun and less desirable as a friend, playmate, seatmate, classmate, and neighbor than the nonsuckers.

So if buckteeth aren't bad enough, social ostracism is yet another reason to quit the thumb.

What is that thing hanging down in the back of your throat, and what is it for?

We mentioned that lovely fleshy thing in the back of your throat earlier when we described how milk comes flying from your nose when you laugh. It's called the uvula, from the Latin word *uva*, which means grape. If you take a look in the mirror, you will notice that this skin flap is shaped like a tear or a grape. If yours has a little fish tail, don't panic, that's called a bifid uvula and it's not a problem at all.

The uvula is an interesting little thing. The uvula has its own little muscle, the muscularis uvula, which allows it to move and change shape. This prevents food from going down the wrong way, and it also has a minor role in speech. Some singers believe the uvula helps them produce a vibrato.

Don't worry if your uvula is swollen. Many things can cause this including: tonsillitis, viral infections of the throat, allergies, or trauma.

If you are passing through Los Angeles, Billy can introduce you to his close friend who will be happy to show you that he has no uvula. No, he wasn't maimed at birth, it was removed in a procedure called a uvulopalatopharyngoplasty. Try saying that five times fast. Removal of the uvula is performed as a treatment for sleep apnea or excessive snoring.

Why do your ears pop in an airplane?

We are now making our final approach into the end of this chapter. Please put your seat backs and tray tables in an upright and locked position ... We couldn't resist. We always wanted to give that speech.

When you take off in an airplane, the air pressure decreases as you ascend. The air trapped in your inner ear needs to escape and equalize the pressure between your inner ear and the atmosphere. The air escapes through the eustachian tube, a small passage between the inner ear and back of the nose/throat. This equalization of pressure is that pop you feel. The same thing happens when landing, but in this case, air pressure increases and air needs to get into the inner ear where the pressure has adjusted to the lower pressure during flight.

You can help your ears to equalize by swallowing, yawning, or chewing. All these aid in the opening of the eustachian tubes. If these don't work, pinch your nostrils shut, take a mouthful of air, and blow. Decongestants and some nasal sprays also help ease the passage of air, especially if you are already congested.

Chapter 7

Women Want to Know

We had finished a long morning of patients and Leyner had taken our receptionist, Wendy, out to lunch. I was catching up on paperwork when I realized that several hours had passed since they'd left. I called his cell phone, but when I heard Leyner's signature ringtone, the theme from *Popeye*, emanating from his bag in the office, I realized I was out of luck. I continued reviewing charts until I heard a loud and continuous thumping coming from the outer office. I opened the door to find Leyner and Wendy playing hopscotch on a board that Leyner had painted on the carpet with correction fluid.

A drunken Leyner tripped over a floor lamp and after a graceful somersault landed at my feet. "My brother, you missed a glorious celebration, a Dionysian blow-out of epic proportions, a bad-assed bacchanalia fit for the

likes of Caligula and Kim Jong-il and Kate Moss ...
and ..." Leyner seemed to pass out momentarily. Then
his eyes fluttered open. "I think I just had a petit mal
seizure," he said. "It was awesome." Leyner began crawling around on his hands and knees. Soon Wendy was on
the floor with him, making a high-pitched orgasmic
sound.

I got down on my own hands and knees and crawled
toward Leyner. Worried that I had forgotten some special occasion, I whispered into his ear, "Did I forget
Wendy's birthday or something?"

Leyner reared up. "No, it's nobody's birthday ...
Today's February fourth ... C'mon, Professor, don't you
know what that means?"

I looked at him blankly.

"You call yourself an intellectual, a ... doctor?!" he
sneered. "How could you be so insensitive to women?"

I still had no idea what he was getting at.

"Wendy has a lot of female questions she wants to ask
you but first you need a little refresher in the annals of
gynecology. Fifty-five years ago today in Chicago, skilled
surgeons removed a three-hundred-and-eight-pound
ovarian cyst from Gertrude Levandowski and it only
took them ninety-six hours."

"How could I have forgotten?" I said.

Wendy stumbled across the office.

"How much did she drink?" I asked, having never
seen Wendy intoxicated in the least, never mind three
sheets to the wind.

"Seven or eight whiskey sours, I think. I outran her

two to one … Anyhow, in honor of the day she's become very inquisitive about … uh …" Leyner cleared his throat. "About her … cycles … and her … infrastructure."

Wendy perked up and stared at me with an unfocused look. "Can I trust you?"

Not knowing what was about to come, I replied, "Of course, Wendy. Anything you ask I will hold in my strictest confidence."

Leyner stood erect and gave a crisp military salute. "What happens in Vegas stays in Vegas."

"Okay, then." She took a deep breath. "Please tell me. I have to know." She hiccupped. "Is there danger that if I watch *Herbie Fully Loaded* too many times, that I will … synchronize my period with Lindsay Lohan?"

With that, she and Leyner passed out in perfect unison.

Why do women always get urinary-tract infections?

Many women are familiar with the symptoms of a urinary-tract infection or UTI. It usually starts with a persistent urge to urinate or a burning sensation when you pee. You also can have blood in the urine, cloudy, strong-smelling urine, or pain in the lower part of your abdomen. About 50 percent of women will have a urinary-tract infection at some time during their lives. The female-to-male ratio for urinary tract infections is about thirty to one.

Why are women so blessed with this uncomfortable gift while men are spared?

Everyone's urine is sterile and meant to stay that way. The difference between women and men begins with the urethra, the tube through which urine leaves the body. The urethra is shorter in women than in men, thus making it easier for bacteria to travel the wrong way up this one-way street. The urethra also is located closer to the rectum in women, and there are more bacteria in this area that can find their way into the bladder. Sexual activity can also push bacteria into the sterile urine.

The medical term for bladder infections is cystitis. If there is a lot of blood with a urine infection, we call it hemorrhagic cystitis. There's even a special variety, "honeymoon cystitis," which refers to the urine infections that women get on their honeymoon from frequent and prolonged sexual intercourse.

Luckily, there are some ways to help prevent urinary-tract infections. Women should always urinate after sexual intercourse, wipe themselves from front to back, and empty their bladders fully when they go to the bathroom. Proving once again that a woman's work is never done. Men only tend to get their infections when they are older as the prostate grows and causes a blockage of the urinary flow.

What is that sound a vagina makes after sex?

This is definitely an embarrassing question to both ask and answer, but we'll give it a shot.

The sound occurs when air gets pushed into the vagina during sexual intercourse. After sex, when the penis is removed, air is released and you get some vaginal flatulence. "Queef" and "vart" are two colorful slang terms that are used to describe these noises that a woman may emit after sex. These sounds are perfectly normal, so there is nothing to worry about.

Are fat women more fertile?

The best way to answer this question is to refer back to one of our favorite childhood fairy tales, "Goldilocks and the Three Bears." Remember when sweet little Goldilocks was looking for a bed to sleep in and she found one that was "too soft," one that was "too hard," and, yes, ultimately one that was "just right"? The same goes for this question. Both obesity and extreme thinness can be associated with infertility. You need to be "just right" to conceive easily.

There are several reasons why very high or very low body fat can affect fertility. Fat tissue is involved in converting androgens (male hormones) to estrogen. Since body fat is a significant source of estrogen, it would seem logical to think that more body fat means more hormones and that that would be a good thing. Well, fertility requires a fine balance, and it really depends on the type of hormones that are around. If you are too thin, you make a form of estrogen that is too weak, but if you are too fat, the higher level of estrogen sends signals to the brain that affect your ability to stimulate the formation of eggs.

Now, we need to clarify exactly what "fat" means. In our society, there are crazy definitions of fat and thin. Magazines are littered with starving actresses and models who are thought to exemplify the ideal weight. Let us try to stop the insanity.

Body mass index (BMI) is a reliable indicator of total body fat and is the most commonly used measurement related to the risk of disease and death. It is calculated using the formula, $BMI = kg/m^2$. Sound hard? There are many online calculators where you simply enter your weight and height and get your BMI. The score works for both men and women, but it does have some limitations. BMI may overestimate body fat in athletes or people who have a very muscular build. It also can underestimate body fat in older persons and those who have lost muscle mass. In general, a body mass index between nineteen and thirty will keep you in the right range to have normal reproductive ability.

Are top and bottom herpes the same thing?

Herpes is everywhere. Yes, we said it, but don't panic. There is no need to duct-tape your doors and windows, wear surgical gloves, or cover your home toilet seat with one of those paper rings. We just want to break the herpes stigma.

Herpes viruses are extremely common and rank just behind influenza and cold viruses in frequency. Chicken-pox virus, shingles, and mononucleosis all are caused by members of the herpes family. And then there are the two most famous herpes viruses, Herpes simplex virus 1 (HSV-1) and Herpes simplex virus 2 (HSV-2).

HSV-1 and HSV-2 are virtually identical under the microscope. Herpes simplex virus 1, or "top herpes," is usually associated with infections of the lips, mouth, and face. HSV-1 causes cold sores (or fever blisters) and is transmitted by contact with infected saliva. Herpes 2 or "bottom herpes" is sexually transmitted. This type is responsible for genital herpes. Despite these generalities, either type can reside in either or both parts of the body.

By the time you are an adult, about 90 percent of people will have antibodies to HSV-1. On the other hand, only 30 percent of adults in the United States have antibodies against HSV-2. Luckily, many who are infected have almost no symptoms. Cross-infection of type 1 and 2 viruses can occur from oral-genital contact.

Can friends synchronize their menstrual cycles?

Oh my! We had no idea that we needed a PhD in statistics to read about this topic. There has been about thirty years of research about the possibility that women who spend a lot of time together can synchronize their menstrual cycles. We invite you to delve into the annals of research on estrous synchrony or menstrual synchrony yourself and read about the controversy surrounding this topic. It is exciting stuff!

In 1971, Martha McClintock, a psychologist, published a paper that first reported this phenomenon. Since then, many scientists and statisticians have investigated the possibility and haven't found any link. There is no physiological explanation as to why this happens. But, based on statistical analysis—in other words, simply by sheer coincidence—some overlap of periods can be expected in any group of friends.

Why can you eat three times more than normal when you have PMS?

When we looked into food cravings *during* menstrual periods, we weren't able to find any scientific cause. Premenstrual gluttony (lovely term, we know), on the other hand, has an explanation.

Imagine the cycle divided in half, with the time of ovulation being the midpoint. The first half is called the follicular phase and the second half, the luteal. Studies in baboons, Rhesus monkeys, and pigtail monkeys have shown increased food intake in the premenstrual period, or the luteal phase of the menstrual cycle. In humans, food intake has also been observed to be highest in the luteal phase. It is not entirely clear why this happens, but researchers think it has to do with changes in serotonin levels during the menstrual cycle that make you crave more food.

Is your waist twice the size of your neck?

Anthropometry is the study of human body measurement for use in anthropological classification and comparison. What fun! Let's whip out those tape measures and calipers!

There is a lot of research out there, so prepare yourself if you're going to explore this area. Unfortunately, I sat down in my kitchen to do the research and before I knew it, four hours had passed and I had made my way through a box of Gummy Bears, two Twix bars, a jar of peanuts, and a leftover roast-beef sandwich. Now my waist and neck are the same size and I can barely reach the keyboard, but I am prepared to pass on some information.

Our editor was the inquiring mind who asked this one, and unfortunately, there is only one nonmedical mention that relates directly to the comparison between neck and waist size. Apparently, in dressmakers' guidelines from the turn of the century, a girl's eligibility was said to be judged by the size of her waist—which should be "twice the circumference of her neck, which, in turn, should be twice the circumference of her wrist."

The medical literature has many references to both waist circumference and neck circumference, but they do not address any direct correlation in size. According to the National Institutes of Health, a high waist circumference is associated with an increased risk for type 2 diabetes, high cholesterol, high blood pressure, and heart disease. A British study showed that over the past fifty years, waist measurements alone have increased by 6.5 inches in women. Neck circumference has also been linked to increased heart disease, diabetes, and sleep apnea risk.

Before we leave the topic of body size behind, we have to mention one article from the November 1995 *International Journal of Eating Disorders*. In their article "Distorting Reality for Children: Body Size Proportions of Barbie and Ken Dolls," K. D. Brownell and M. A. Napolitano used hip measurements as a constant, and calculated the changes necessary for a young, healthy adult woman and man to attain the same body proportions as Barbie and Ken. Among the changes necessary were for the female to increase 24 inches in height, 5 inches in the chest, and 3.2 inches in neck length, while decreasing 6 inches in the waist. Male Ken wannabes need to increase 20 inches in height, 11 inches in the chest, and 7.9 inches in neck circumference. If Barbie were a real female, she would be 7 feet 2 inches with a 22-inch waist and a neck that could barely support her head. Ken would be 7 feet 8 inches with a 43-inch waist. A little unrealistic, no?

Why do your boobs get tender before your period?

Some breast pain before your period is perfectly normal. Hormonal fluctuations cause changes in the breast ducts and the breast lobules. The lobules are the milk-producing tissues of the breast. Each breast has about fifteen to twenty lobes that branch into smaller lobules, and each lobule ends in a bulb. Milk originates in the bulbs and is carried by ducts to the nipple.

The boob pain usually starts during the second half of the menstrual cycle. When estrogen production increases and peaks just prior to the middle of your cycle, it causes enlargement of the breast ducts. Then, right before your period, another hormone (progesterone) peaks and causes growth of the breast lobules. These increases in size lead to pain.

Premenstrual breast pain can be mild or severe. Pain is usually less acute in women who are taking birth-control pills. Some women find that caffeine intake can increase breast pain during that time. Simple anti-inflammatory medications can reduce the pain. Also avoid very aggressive teenage boys who want to feel you up but haven't yet learned the correct method.

Why don't women have hairy chests?

Well, actually some women do.

As a culture, we are obsessed with becoming hairless. There are waxing salons, threading salons, laser hair-removal treatments, and electrolysis. The truth is that as mammals we are designed to be covered in body hair. We have the same number of hair follicles as our hairier simian friends, but our hair is shorter and finer. The only truly hairless parts of the body are the umbilicus (belly button), the lips, the nipples, the palms, and the soles.

There are two types of hair on the body, vellus hair and terminal hair. Vellus hair is soft, fine, colorless, and short. Vellus hair helps the body maintain a steady temperature by providing some insulation. Terminal hair is found on the head, the armpits, and the pubic area, and on the face and chest in males. It is coarser, darker, and longer than vellus hair.

Hirsutism is the growth of long, coarse hair on the face and body of a woman in a pattern similar to men. Hirsutism can be the result of many medical conditions including polycystic ovary syndrome, hormonal imbalance, tumors, thyroid disease, obesity, anorexia, or medications. Excess hair on the face or chest may simply be due to your genetics. Luckily, there are plenty of ways to get rid of excess hair.

2:05 p.m.

Gberg: Leyner?

Gberg: I need your hirsute help.

Leyner: Are you making fun of my back hair?

Gberg: I would never mock your back hair, but I would occasionally recommend a grooming of your neck.

Leyner: Just got manscaped the other day ... you haven't seen me since.

Gberg: Manscaped?

Leyner: Haircut ... the works.

Gberg: That is fantastic.

Leyner: That word ...?

Leyner: Learned it from Gabs or Mercedes ... I used it in my eyebrow-shaving answer.

Gberg: Yes. I had never heard it before.

Leyner: Me either ... isn't it great?!

Gberg: I am answering the question on "Why don't women have hairy chests?" and I know you are the evolutionary expert of the two of us.

Leyner: Hmmmm ...

2:10 p.m.

Gberg: I have the *Naked Ape* book that my brother gave me, but I thought I would take a shortcut and seek your sage advice.

Leyner: Humans did reach some wonderful mutation somewhere along the road to the present ... that resulted in uniquely large and hairless breasts for our females.

Leyner: Let me check something I printed out ... hold on.

Gberg: Well, not entirely hairless. There is that layer of almost invisible fur.

Leyner: That's "down."

Leyner: That's what keeps women from being confused for porcelain figurines.

Gberg: Is that a hip-hop expression or are you

talking about vellus hair?

Leyner: Vellus hair ... sounds like a salon.

Gberg: We should open a salon. You could be like Warren Beatty in *Shampoo*.

2:15 p.m.

Leyner: Have you read "Breast Asymmetry, Sexual, and Human Reproductive Success" by Anders Pape Moller of the Zoological Institute in Copenhagen?

Gberg: No, have you read "The Hairlessness Norm: The Removal of Body Hair in Women"?

Leyner: I'd love to read it. Print one out for me. I'll stick in a copy of *Anna Karenina* so I can pretend to be reading Tolstoy on the subway, when I'm actually reading about the axillary hair of women throughout history.

Gberg: I have found some great articles this time around.

2:20 p.m.

Gberg: Here is another one for you to read on the train ... "Body Hair Scores and Total Hair Diameters in Healthy Women in the Kirikkale Region of Turkey."

Leyner: I'm not sure I'd risk reading that one on the PATH ... I don't want to have the soles of my feet beaten by some enraged Turk.

Leyner: I think women's body hair is sexy ... but not chest hair.

Gberg: I am surprised, you seem to be somewhat pugilistic when traveling underground.

Leyner: My uncle Fred used to tell me (when I was a wee little lad) that potato salad made hair grow on your chest ...

Leyner: I'm most alive the farther down I go.

Gberg: Yeah, what was with that "it puts hair on your chest" line?

Leyner: You had an Uncle Fred too????!!!!

Gberg: As we are becoming more hairless, the line will probably reverse itself and you will see a macho guy drinking moonshine and saying "It takes hair off your chest!"

2:25 p.m.

Leyner: It was some piece of old folkloric aphoristic wisdom ... do this or do that and it'll put hair on your chest. Shot of whiskey, spoonful of castor oil, half-pound of potato salad ...

Leyner: Body hair does seem to have an important evolutionary function ...

Leyner: But I can't tell you what it is ... cause it'll give away my brilliant 208-page response to the question: Why Do We Have Pubic Hair?

Gberg: We need an evolutionary biologist as a co-author.

Gberg: They could do all the waxing in the salon we open.

Leyner: I'd say that evolutionary biology is just

speculative enough that I can qualify as an expert.

Leyner: I think women are becoming too hairless.

Gberg: You are the expert of all experts. Who else uses the word aphoristic in an IM?

Leyner: Thank you.

Gberg: *De nada.*

Gberg: I disagree. I suffer from hirsutophobia.

Leyner: I know ... you need to deal with that.

Gberg: I totally made up that word but it turns out to be a real one.

Leyner: Don't certain apes have hairless chests?

Leyner: How's about trichomania?

Gberg: Baboons have those red hairless butts. What an evolutionary kick in the pants!

2:30 p.m.

Leyner: That's the species that anal-bleaching was invented for, see?

Gberg: Must you come back to that again.

Leyner: Couldn't help it. Look, if we're going to open a salon ... we need to offer a FULL range of services ...

Gberg: What goes around, comes around.

Leyner: Manicures, pedicures, facials, waxing, and anal bleaching.

Leyner: And if a woman comes in and needs her chest waxed ... and you're to squeamish to do it ... I will.

Leyner: Too squeamish—sorry.

Leyner: I got too indignant to type.

Gberg: I am. I will leave that to you. And the biologist.

Leyner: Who thought it would come to this ... that I'd end up a fraudulent evolutionary biologist who owns a chest waxing/anal bleaching salon?

2:35 p.m.

Gberg: A fitting last hurrah.

Gberg: All right, I need to get back to the hairy chest question. Onward and upward.

Leyner: Here's to the generative powers of good potato salad, comrade.

Leyner: Victory or death!

Gberg: Hallelulah.

Leyner: Ciao, baby.

Gberg: Adios.

Do women have wet dreams?

Sorry, Virginia, there is no Santa Claus, but women can have wet dreams or, more specifically, nocturnal orgasms—and that may be better than finding a new cashmere sweater under your tree.

Alfred Kinsey, the famous sex researcher, found that nocturnal orgasms were reported by 90 percent of the men, but by less than 40 percent of the women in his studies. So common are male wet dreams that the Bible has several references to male nocturnal emissions. It doesn't, however, specifically address female nocturnal orgasms. Now we don't want to create a biblical argument on the topic, so we will leave it for you to interpret.

If there be among you any man, that is not clean by reason of uncleanness that chanceth him by night, then shall he go abroad out of the camp, he shall not come within the camp.

—Deuteronomy 23:10

And if a man has an emission of semen, he shall bathe his whole body in water, and be unclean until the evening. And every garment and every skin on which the semen comes shall be washed with water, and be unclean until the evening. If a man lies with a woman and has an emission of semen, both of them shall bathe themselves in water and be unclean until the evening.

—Leviticus 15:16–18

Amen.

Is douching dangerous?

Leyner and I both clearly remember the American airwaves being pounded with douche advertising in the 1980s. How can you forget the image of a daughter asking her mother if she ever gets that "not so fresh feeling" and then proceeds to flush herself with a vinegar and water solution. It always made us think of someone giving themselves an enema with salad dressing.

These ads are less visible now, but some companies are still selling these products. But there is no evidence that these products are necessary, and actually, the very practice of vaginal douching may be dangerous.

Vaginal douching has been around for centuries and evolved at a time when there were no medications to treat infections. It involves flushing a special solution (usually water and vinegar) into the vagina under the premise that it flushes out bacteria to reduce or eliminate odor. Vaginal douching has many risks and has been linked to a number of adverse health conditions, including bacterial and yeast infections, pelvic inflammatory disease (PID), ectopic pregnancy, preterm birth, reduced fertility, and increased susceptibility to sexually transmitted diseases.

Remember, there is no need to use any fancy grooming products; the vagina is a self-cleaning oven.

Is there a treatment for severe PMS?

This is no joke (but it probably won't stop us from making one later). PMS is real and it can be severe.

Here is something from the DSM-IV (*Diagnostic and Statistical Manual of Mental Disorders*), where a severe form of PMS is listed as a "Depressive Disorder Not Otherwise Specified":

Premenstrual dysphoric disorder: in most menstrual cycles during the past year, symptoms (e.g., markedly depressed mood, marked anxiety, marked affective lability, decreased interest in activities) regularly occurred during the last week of the luteal phase (and remitted within a few days of the onset of menses). These symptoms must be severe enough to markedly interfere with work, school, or usual activities and be entirely absent for at least one week postmenses.

Now, this is much more serious than your wife yelling at you for not taking out the garbage.

Premenstrual dysphoric disorder (PMDD) affects around 3 to 8 percent of women during their reproductive years. Exactly what causes it is not fully understood, but the sequence of events begins with ovulation, which triggers a series of changes in neurotransmitters. The most important of these is serotonin, and a reduction in serotonin has been found in the second half of the menstrual cycle. There have been many medical studies on this topic and there are many different treatment options. The most effective approaches are the use of drugs that either block serotonin reuptake (antidepressants) or suppress ovulation (birth-control pills). Other options include exercise, which helps increase endorphins,

Vitamin B$_6$, dietary changes including reduced caffeine and increased complex carbohydrates, and *Vitex agnus-castus* extract Ze 440 (chaste berry fruit).

Is depression more common in women?

Most investigators report that depression is twice as common in women when compared with men. This holds true in the United States and in many societies around the world. For major depression, this ratio approaches almost three in one. It is estimated that nearly 340 million people worldwide and 18 million people in the United States suffer from depression.

There are several explanations for the disproportionate rate of depression in women. Hormonal changes around the time of pregnancy, menopause, and the premenstrual period can cause mood disturbances. Sexual or physical abuse is also more common in women and may contribute to higher rates of depression. It is also believed that women are more likely than men to talk about their symptoms and admit feelings of depression.

The last explanation comes from our wives. They argue that a woman is bound to be depressed when she has to put up with men who never listen; talk incessantly about sex, poop, and sports; and obsessively babble on about some book they wrote.

• Chapter 8 •

A Funny Thing Happened on the Way to the Spa

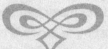

I was in a particularly great mood walking into the office one day as I bounced through the door, whistling. Crossing through the doorway, I noticed a bizarre odor in the waiting room and I saw Wendy with a bandanna covering her mouth and nose frantically spraying air freshener. Her eyes were watering uncontrollably and she pointed toward the office, shaking her head. I took a deep breath, coughed, and opened the door. I then came upon the most harrowing sight. Leyner was seated in the corner of the office, semiconscious, one eye crusted shut, his hair matted and clumped, an unidentifiable layer of some cheesy material coating his upper torso. There was a sickening stench emanating from his direction that made it physically perilous to get any closer to him. I'd become used to Leyner's eccentricities and bizarre behaviour, but this was a new dimension. He'd always been somewhat vain about his physical allure … something extreme surely must have happened. Holding a dampened handkerchief to my mouth and nose, I approached Leyner and shook him gently. "What happened? Tell me."

Leyner's crusted eye opened with an audible crackle.

"I met a bunch of exiled Japanese gangster hit men playing miniature golf …"

"What? How do you know they were exiled Japanese gangster hit men?"

"They were really, really, REALLY good miniature-golf players, first of all … and none of them had pinkies."

"And … ?"

"So we meet this bunch of girls … grad students from Rensselaer Polytech … and they seem out for some fun and games. And one of the gangster guys says in a guttural tone, 'It is an honored tradition for you to pick one of us. The handsomest one.' We all paraded in front of them … And I'm thinking, there's no contest here … first of all, I have both my pinkies. Second … I don't know … I just think I'm a pretty hot kinda hunky guy … don't you?"

As lost and decrepit as Leyner was at the moment, there was no way I could do anything but nod.

"So they rate us … like pieces of meat … and … and …" Leyner's head fell despondently. "And I came in … last."

I didn't know quite what to say. For Leyner to have been rated worst-in-show among a motley crew of maimed miniature golfers must have been devastating.

I tried to reassure my partner. "Leyner, why do you care what a bunch of knock-kneed engineering students think? Maybe they just prefer Asian men."

Leyner wasn't soothed at all. "That was my first reaction, but then when I suggested that, the Japanese gangster took great offense and tossed me in the Dumpster behind the concession stand. I was so mortified that I took a sleeping tablet and slept in a pool of fryer grease and discarded nacho cheese."

Leyner seemed to have lost some of his normal bravado.

Dejectedly, he added, "I guess it's hard to realize that I've finally lost my mojo."

In a moment of surprising candor, Leyner looked up at me and said, "You're a doctor, help me!"

My mind raced through a list of pharmaceuticals, but I imagined Leyner abusing them all. Then I realized a simple solution. "Leyner you don't need a doctor."

"I don't," he said with a glimmer of hope.

"No, you just need a makeover!"

Wendy, who obviously had been listening with her ear pressed to the door, was at our sides in a second. "I know just the place to start."

Two minutes later, we were in front of the local firehouse where Wendy had charmed several firefighters into hosing Leyner down with their most powerful water cannon.

"It's exfoliating!!" yelled Wendy as Leyner was blasted against a wall by the force of the water.

From there we patronized a dizzying series of Manhattan's most prestigious grooming establishments.

Plucked, massaged, manicured, tanned, conditioned, waxed, coiffed, and moisturized, Leyner emerged a radiant and resplendent thing of beauty.

"You're magnificent!!" Wendy exclaimed.

Leyner smiled and with a look of determination in his eyes turned and began walking off.

"Where are you going?" I asked.

"Troy, baby, Troy."

I was baffled by Leyner's mythological reference. Was he making some esoteric allusion to *The Iliad*?

Leyner sensed my confusion, smirked, and added, "Troy, New York—the home of Rensselaer Polytech!"

I instantly realized that the old, irrepressible, irredeemably narcissistic Leyner was back.

Why do I sneeze when I pluck my eyebrows?

Duh … that's so obvious. Just kidding. What could possibly be the connection between a tweezed eyebrow hair and a sneeze?

The sneezing reflex is a complex chain reaction of physiological events. It typically starts with an irritation to your nasal passages that excites your trigeminal nerve. (No, it doesn't take much to get a trigeminal nerve excited.) Then these impulses are transmitted through the trigeminal ganglion to a set of neurons in the brain stem called the sneezing center. The sneezing center then sends impulses back along the facial nerve to your nasal passages, mucus glands, blood vessels, and eyelids, which is the reason you close your eyes when you sneeze. (Impulses from the sneezing center also travel to nerves that control muscles in your abdomen, chest, diaphragm, and neck.)

Plucking a hair from your eyebrow stimulates a nearby branch of the nerve that services your nasal passages. And even though these impulses don't originate in your nose, the eyebrow-plucking sensitizes the entire nerve, enabling sufficient impulses to reach the sneezing center … and you sternutate (that's sneeze, in dorky doctor-speak, remember).

So whether you're shaping those ultra-feminine crescents or manscaping that unibrow, here's a hearty "Gusundheit!" for the next time you pluck.

Can deodorant really cause breast cancer?

For several years, rumors have circulated, primarily on the Internet, claiming that the use of antiperspirant deodorants can cause breast cancer. But no clear scientific basis has been found to substantiate these rumors.

According to the National Cancer Institute, "Researchers at the NCI are not aware of any conclusive evidence linking the use of underarm antiperspirants or deodorants and the subsequent development of breast cancer. The U.S. Food and Drug Administration, which regulates food, cosmetics, medicines, and medical devices, also does not have any evidence or research data that ingredients in underarm antiperspirants or deodorants cause cancer."

These rumors have two basic premises. They claim that antiperspirants (because they block perspiration) prevent the body from flushing "toxins," which then accumulate in the lymph nodes of the armpits and cause cancer. Other reports speculate that potentially harmful ingredients in some of these products, including a group of chemicals called parabens, might enter the body through nicks caused by under-arm shaving and cause breast cancer.

A small study did find parabens in eighteen of twenty samples of breast-cancer tissue. But since the study failed to establish whether the samples were from women who used deodorants or antiperspirants containing parabens, or even the source of the parabens in the samples (parabens are present in a variety of foods, medicines, and cosmetics)—it certainly doesn't provide proof of any relevant hypothesis.

A recent study involving breast-cancer survivors found that women who used underarm antiperspirants/deodorants and shaved their underarms frequently were diagnosed with cancer at younger ages, but the study stopped short of showing a clear link.

In 2002, a study was conducted at the Fred Hutchinson Cancer Research Center in Seattle. This research, which involved some 1,606 women—813 with breast cancer, and 793 controls—indicated no relationship between breast cancer and use of either an antiperspirant or a deodorant.

Why do women's toes curl after years of wearing high heels?

The torments women will endure in the name of glamour! Never mind the fact that when you're wearing high heels, you actually have to realign your spine so you don't fall over. Or the fact that a research team at Harvard University found a link between high heels and knee osteoarthritis, a degenerative joint disease. Or the fact that they can shorten your Achilles tendon and cause something called metatarsalgia—chronic pain in the ball of the foot.

Let's just focus on those toes for a moment. Do you want a bunion (a painful inflammation of bone and tissue on the side of your big or little toe)? Wear heels. How do hammertoes sound? Hammertoes is a permanent foot deformity. When you crunch and crowd those poor toes of yours into a narrow shoe and clench them to grasp the shoe, over time the tendons in your toes will curl up and stiffen into a claw-like shape or a … hammer. Who needs DIY stores, when you can transform your own appendages into tools?

Granted, there's a mutual fantasy in the world of high heels. Wearing heels makes women feel sexier, and men love leering at hotties navigating the city in their stilettos. And for every Manolo-shod woman who dreams of being Carrie Bradshaw, there's some haggard straphanger out there whose inner Mr. Big is just waiting to emerge. But until men trade their flats for 4-inch spiked heels, it's women, and women alone, who'll bear the brunt of the pain.

Why does your skin get so dry in the winter?

Winter is rough enough with the snow and the sleet and the hacking away at ice-encrusted windshields in the dark, frigid mornings. But that dry, chapped, cracked skin just adds insult to injury … or is it injury to insult?

Because the relative humidity—moisture in the air—gets so low in the cold season, winter weather dries out our skin. And there's not much relief to be found inside—indoor heating also lowers humidity, depriving the skin of moisture. In the cold weather, many of us develop something commonly called "winter itch" or xerotic eczema—dry, itchy, flaky skin. To help cope, dermatologists have three words for you: moisturize, moisturize, moisturize.

Apply moisturizers to your skin right after you get out of the bath or shower. And don't bathe or shower too frequently. Exposure to hot water can actually further dehydrate your skin, and detergent-based soaps and cleansers can remove the skin's natural moisturizers. Also, you might want to consider purchasing a humidifier.

And, if all else fails, you can always just pack up and move to Maui.

Is it true that hair grows back thicker after shaving?

No. And if this were true, wouldn't women who've shaved for years have legs and armpits like gorillas?

One of the reasons for this common misperception may be that new-grown stubble seems thicker than uncut hair. But the truth is, all hair growth takes place below the skin, down in the hair follicle. The section of the hair we lop off is just dead protein.

Shaving doesn't make your hair grow back any faster or thicker or darker or coarser.

If there were even the slightest chance that shaving caused thicker regrowth, men suffering from male-pattern baldness would be hacking away at their shiny pates with the latest five-bladed razor from dawn till dusk.

What causes ingrown hairs?

Oh, you must mean pseudofolliculitis barbae. C'mon, wouldn't you rather have pseudofolliculitis barbae (PFB) than "ingrown hairs" or "razor bumps"? (If this reminds you of a traditional Italian song, you're thinking of "Funiculi, Funicula," which refers to a funicular railway, a kind of mountainside cable car, and has nothing to do with ingrown hairs or razor bumps.)

All these terms refer to basically the same condition, which occurs when the end of a hair shaft is cut, giving it a sharpened edge, and that hair shaft, as it grows, curls, either piercing the adjacent skin or a hair follicle. (This would be your extrafollicular penetration or your transfollicular penetration.) Either can cause a foreign-body inflammatory response and infection. PFB is frequently the result of shaving, hence the term "razor bumps." And the condition is more common in people with curly hair. (It affects some 60 percent of African American men.)

Obviously, people who have to shave each and

every day would be especially likely to contract PFB. And who has to shave every single day, like it or not? Men in the military. (Here's a cheerful grooming tip from a recent issue of *Military Medicine* magazine: "The combat environment, with the recent threat of biological and chemical weapons, requires the servicemen to be clean-shaven for appropriate gas mask fitting around the face.")

So the military has actually developed and implemented a written PFB Treatment Protocol. No, it's not "Don't Shave, Don't Tell." It's more like "Sir, request permission to totally avoid shaving for three to four weeks until all lesions have subsided, while applying Vioform-HC cream each morning; and to soften whiskers, begin a nightly application of Retin-A Cream 0.05 to 0.1% to beard skin while beard is growing out; and implement a circular brushing of the beard area with a polyester skin-cleaning pad or medium-firm toothbrush, four times a day for three to five minutes; and, once shaving bumps subside, to avoid a close shave by water-softening beard first with a hot, wet washcloth for five minutes, and then using a lubricating shaving gel and a PFB razor, and shaving with the grain of the beard, not stretching the skin, and using only one stroke over each area of the beard. Sir!"

10:02 a.m.

Gberg: *¿Que pasa, amigo?*

Leyner: Working on our latest blockbuster ... finishing up A Funny Thing Happened on the Way to the Spa today ...

Leyner: Just reviewing a 25-page document.

Leyner: The navy's protocol for handling pseudofolliculitis barbae.

Gberg: I am deep in the research myself. Reading an article, "Humor, Laughter, and Physical Health: Methodological Issues and Research Findings."

Leyner: Does that include dark, misanthropic laughter?

Gberg: No solid evidence. but I might start wearing a beanie with a propeller on it to work.

Gberg: Absolutely.

Leyner: The health benefits of schadenfreude, etc.

10:05 a.m.

Leyner: And schnitzel.

Gberg: You know my thoughts. Happy complaining.

Gberg: Spaetzle-those German dumplings.

Leyner: I was just about to type that ... but I hesitated at the spelling ... damn!

Gberg: He who types first types ...

Leyner: There's a new place we should try ... where the ol' Le Zinc used to be.

Gberg: Siegried's Spaetzle House.

Leyner: German ... nice spaetzle, I bet ... but ...

Leyner: Probably not so good in the chubby, horny German waitress department.

Gberg: You were the head of that department in your last job, weren't you?

Leyner: Weird fantasy of mine ... sort of lonely PTA mom/beer maid.

Leyner: Yes!

Gberg: You are watching too much Heidi Klum on *Project Runway*.

Leyner: I also did postdoctoral work in chubby, horny German waitresses in 19th-Century American Poetry.

10:10 a.m.

Gberg: I am at a loss. I have a cold and lack the energy to respond to your Leynerisms.

Gberg: I can't believe that this time next week we will have a baby.

Gberg: Not we meaning me and you but we meaning me and Jessica.

Leyner: Yes, we'll have our baby, darling.

Leyner: I feel like I'm in some soap opera right now.

Gberg: I am talking about my impending fatherhood.

Gberg: I am hormonal and I need attention.

Leyner: No no no, it's just the IM delay ... PLEASE! Don't take it so hard, bitch!

Leyner: I know ... I know ... relax ... breathe ... breathe ...

Gberg: Like in LeMans class.

Gberg: It always makes me think of pregnant race-car drivers.

Leyner: One of the nun/nurses at the hospital in which Gabs was born told Mercedes ... after Merci moaned a bit ... she said ... "Why do you think they call it labor, sweetheart?"

10:15 a.m.

Leyner: I like freaky Japanese motocross stars, myself.

Gberg: Who was that Lamaze guy anyway? Some French doctor who got the world panting.

Leyner: Next life, that's what I'm doing. I want to be a Japanese motocross champion.

Gberg: Did you see the snowboard cross in the Olympics?

Gberg: I think they should combine that with short-track speed skating and create a bad-ass biathalon.

Leyner: Good question ... Lamaze ...

Leyner: They should have a sport that combines snowboarding, shooting your friend in the face with bird shot, and giving birth.

Gberg: Cheney can coach the second leg, but I can't see him being much help in the snow-boarding or birthing categories.

Leyner: Also ... they should replace the broom in

curling with a vacuum cleaner ... make it much more exciting.

Leyner: Maybe one of those vacuum cleaners that can pick up a bowling ball ...

Gberg: I think we should start our own curling league. Shuffleboard on ice.

Leyner: You'd be surprised at how tender right-wing draft-deferring plutocrats can be when his own baby crowns.

10:20 a.m.

Leyner: Sorry for the bad grammar ... when their own babies crown.

Leyner: Shuffleboard would definitely be in my Olympics ... and mah-jongg ... and senile incompetent driving.

Gberg: And pinochle.

Gberg: My grandfather was a card shark down in Florida.

Leyner: And ill-considered, heedless, insulting remark-spewing.

Leyner: My grandparents played picochle, canasta, and mah-jongg.

Gberg: I can picture you in one of those weight-lifting leotards spewing insults and then assuming a victory pose.

Leyner: And my dad's mom was, like U.S. champion in that game Battleship.

Gberg: "Oh and Leyner really stuck that landing."

Leyner: Nana ...

Gberg: She played competitive Connect Four?

Leyner: I love those incredibly thick weight-lifting belts the enormous Slavic weight lifters wear ...

10:25 a.m.

Gberg: We should have had a question about those belts in the book. For the sports chapter.

Leyner: She also played competitive Rock 'Em, Sock 'Em Robots. She was considered a grand-master at that, actually.

Gberg: Not that I am suggesting that we add any more work to our already voluminous opus.

Leyner: I love all the ritual of competitive weight lifting ... the dipping of the hands in the chalk ...

Leyner: The snort of ammonia ...

Leyner: The explosive protrusion of the bilateral inguinal hernia!!

Gberg: Did you ever see that *Saturday Night Live* with the all-steroid Olympics?

Leyner: No.

Gberg: The weight lifter yanks the bar and rips his arms off.

Leyner: I'm completely unopposed to steroid use in professional athletes. I think it's fine. Just another sacrifice an athlete's willing to make to entertain the crowd, I think.

Gberg: Then the announcers say something like "Oh, that's got to be very disappointing."

Leyner: That's funny ... I saw a video once ... something someone e-mailed me ... of some poor weight lifter suffering a massive prolapse of some sort or another.

Leyner: I think all his internal organs came out his ass.

Gberg: I saw that picture also ... rectal prolapse.

10:30 a.m.

Leyner: They should show that in the schools ... the way they used to show those bloody car-crash films in driving school.

Gberg: That could be our start in the film business.

Gberg: Warning kids about the dangers of straining while weight lifting.

Leyner: You're so ruthless and ambitious for a "healer."

Leyner: I think it's important work.

Leyner: Beats making those public service announcements about how your brain looks like eggs Benedict if you take drugs.

Gberg: Your altruism never ceases to amaze me.

Gberg: Leyner, you are an angel.

Leyner: Oh, you flatter me!!! I'm blushing like a bride on her wedding night.

Gberg: Okay, I need to get back to work.

Leyner: OK, dude. Talk to you later.

Gberg: Later.

Does a calcium deficiency cause rough nails?

There are two facets of our anatomies that are basically dead. (By dead, I mean not sentient, not comprised of living cells, inanimate, *muerto*, y'know … dead.) Our hair and nails. (The parts we cut, shave, and clip.) And yet we seem to spend an inordinate amount of time worrying about these very parts …

Ironic, isn't it? I mean, we don't have bad pancreas days or bad adrenal medulla days … we have bad hair days. And, uh … we don't have Cowper's gland salons, we have nail salons …

If I seem to vamping here a bit, it's because there's a very simple, succinct, and unadorned answer to this question: NO.

Dietary calcium intake has nothing to do with the quality of your fingernails or your toenails. Consuming more calcium will not make your nails less brittle or smoother or grow faster. Nor will it prevent those occasional white spots on the fingernails (which are called "leukonychia," and are usually caused by some long-forgotten injury to the base of the nail or by an allergic reaction to nail polish, and which disappear as the nail grows out).

If you need further proof—c'mon, don't you trust us by now?—peruse the December 14, 2000, issue of *The New England Journal of Medicine*, specifically a study by Dr. Ian R. Reid of the University of Auckland in New Zealand. Dr. Reid's research, involving over 680 women who took either calcium supplements or placebo tablets, showed that there is no correlation between taking calcium supplements and nail quality.

What purpose do freckles serve?

I don't know ... What "purpose" does your butt serve?

Sorry, that was uncalled for. It's just tricky sometimes to discuss things in terms of their "purpose." It becomes a very philosophical question—the teleology of freckles. We can be fairly certain about the evolutionary development of certain traits (like prehensile digits) and discern the advantages and benefits they confer, but when we talk about "purpose" we get into fairly murky territory, because it presupposes some sort of grand plan. What's the "purpose" of poodles, for instance?

A freckle is simply a concentrated deposit of the dark pigment, melanin. Produced by skin cells called melanocytes, melanin helps protect your skin from the ultraviolet (UV) radiation in sunlight. Especially in people with fair complexions—which means that they have less melanin in their skin—exposure to sunlight causes the melanocytes to produce more melanin in these small circular deposits. So people with lighter complexions tend to have more freckles. There are two kinds of freckles: ephelides (which are generally caused by sun exposure and fade in the winter months) and lentigines (which are darker and do not fade in the winter). Heredity is a very important factor when it comes to freckles. Studies have shown that identical twins have an amazing similarity in the actual number of freckles they each have on their bodies. (If you're spending a long, rainy weekend with your identical twin, and you're bored, try counting each other's freckles.)

Now, as far as the "purpose" of a freckly butt— that's something I can probably take a stab at….

Do your eyebrows grow back if shaved?

As any Goth could tell you, if you shave your eyebrows, they grow back. (Actually, only a small percentage of self-described Goths shave their eyebrows. We have no precise statistics on this, but base it on empirical evidence gleaned from friends and family who are themselves Gothic Americans—the term we prefer.)

Remember, all the elements involved in hair growth are in the living part, down in the root. Shaving hair on the head, the face, or any other part of the body leaves that root intact. Shaved eyebrow hair is no exception—it will certainly grow back.

Don't think for a minute that doctors are immune to urban legends and old wives' tales. I was taught, back in medical school, never to shave an eyebrow because it could result in permanent brow alopecia (bald brows). WRONG.

In fact, there was even a study done in 1999 and published in the *Archives of Facial Plastic Surgery*. It was called "Cilia Regrowth of Shaven Eyebrows." We love this study. Five patients had a single brow "randomly" shaven, while the unshaven brow served as a control. The patients were evaluated for brow regrowth during six months and photos were taken. "Two masked observers analyzed the final photographs to determine if they could identify the side that was shaven." Result: all patients had full brow regrowth without any discernable difference between the shaven and unshaven brow. But what's up with the "masked observers"? I guess it gets a little kinky in the lab sometimes.

(Tweezing, by the way, can be a different story. The root of an eyebrow hair is quite sensitive, so if the same hair is plucked again and again, the root can become permanently damaged and eventually the hair may not grow back.)

When you pull out a gray hair, do two come back in its place?

Back in the day, old wives (and old husbands, for that matter) were far too busy eluding predators, fleeing barbarian hordes, and prostrating themselves on the ground in the face of seemingly inexplicable natural phenomena like lightning and eclipses, to come up with patently erroneous tales like this. But today, with your modern conveniences like Sky+, and microwave popcorn, I guess old wives have enough time on their hands to concoct spurious nonsense like this two-gray-hairs-for-each-one-plucked thing.

If you pull out a gray hair, and wait the three months it usually takes for a hair to grow back, and the additional three months it takes for it to get long enough to notice, know what you'll have? One gray hair.

Why don't you get goose bumps on your face?

There seems to be implicit in this question, a kind of longing, a yearning …

Although most of us only get goose bumps on our bodies—primarily our forearms, legs, and backs—some of us actually do get them on our faces.

The language of the goose bump world is rich and poetic. Goose bumps themselves are also known as goose pimples, gooseflesh, and chicken skin. The reflex that produces them is known as horripilation, piloerection, or the pilomotor reflex. Inuits have over 348 different words for goose bumps. (That's not true.)

Goose bumps are caused by tiny muscles at the base of each hair on our bodies, known as arrecotres pilorum, which contract and pull the hair erect. This is a mammalian response to cold (erect hair creates a layer of insulation), although this doesn't work much for people anymore since we've lost most of our body hair. It's also a sympathetic nerve reflex that's related to the flight-or-fight response. A frightened animal's erect hairs might make it appear larger and thus more intimidating to an enemy. This horripilation-as-intimidation technique has become particularly obsolete for us humans. There's nothing like turning yourself into a mass of quivering gooseflesh to intimidate some huge, menacing asshole who's whispering salacious vulgarities into the ear of your date as he drinks your beer.

Anyway … if you really want goose bumps on your face and don't get them, don't try having some skin grafted from your forearm onto your cheek. The odds are against any insurance company reimbursing you for the procedure and it wouldn't work anyway.

Why do some women go bald?

Alopecia—hair loss or baldness—affects some 30 million women in the United States, young and old, according to the American Academy of Dermatology. But hair loss in women is different from male-pattern baldness (androgenic alopecia). For years, scientists believed that the same process was at work in female-pattern baldness as in the male version—a genetically inherited sensitivity to dihydrotestosterone, a by-product of testosterone that can accumulate in and damage the hair follicle. But today, we know that baldness in women can be the result of many factors—there may be a variety of other types of enzymes, as well as hormone receptors and blockers at work.

Hormonal changes following menopause (including changes in the levels of androgens) can produce "female-pattern baldness." Whereas male-pattern baldness usually starts at the temple area or the crown (that bald spot in the back), women more typically have a diffuse thinning around the whole top of the head, with the frontal hairline maintained. But remember—young women, as well as post-menopausal women, can experience hair loss. Other factors in female alopecia can include hormonal changes following pregnancy, and polycystic ovary syndrome (a fairly common hormonal problem in women). There's also alopecia areata—patchy areas of total hair loss caused by an immune disorder—and telogen effluvium—a temporary shedding of hair following childbirth, crash dieting, or surgery. Certain kinds of prescription drugs and chemotherapies can also cause hair loss. There are many possibilities. So the first thing a woman should do if she notices that she's losing hair is to see her doctor and get to the—excuse the pun—root cause.

A lesser known cause of baldness in women is something called trichotillomania (TTM), which is defined, in the venerable *Diagnostic and Statistical Manual of Mental Disorders*, as "the recurrent pulling out of one's hair that results in noticeable hair loss." (Trichotillomania is classified by some clinicians as a form of obsessive-compulsive disorder.) Among adults, TTM is more common among females than among males. A practice related to TTM is called trichophagia, in which the hair is sucked or eaten. And on the most exotic end of the hair-yanking spectrum is Rapunzel syndrome, in which people who eat their hair develop a small or large bowel obstruction caused by a trichobezoar … yes, you guessed it—a hairball.

Does smoking help you lose weight?

There is ample evidence that nicotine does cause an increase in metabolism, and smoking cigarettes may act as an appetite suppressant. The main reason, though, that we tend to associate smoking with weight loss is that people who quit smoking often report gaining some weight. But addiction specialists point out that this is simply because, at first, many ex-smokers use food as a substitute for cigarettes. And, of course, any significant increase in caloric intake without some commensurate calorie-burning exercise will probably result in some added poundage.

But let's be serious here. Even if cigarettes were a

remarkably effective appetite suppressant—which they are NOT—the dangers of smoking are so cata- strophic that only someone with a powerful death wish would actually smoke to lose weight. But maybe fatal lung cancer or emphysema is worth it, consider- ing that morticians are wizards at extreme make- overs, and that embalming fluid does give you a nice sort of glow... .

What makes self-tanner work?

The active ingredient in self-tanners (or "sunless tan- ners," as they're also called) is dihydroxyacetone (DHA). DHA is a colorless sugar that interacts with the amino acid arginine in the dead cells of the stratum corneum, the outermost layer of your epidermis, which is the outer layer of your skin. The interaction of the DHA with these cells in the epidermis causes a color change, a browning of the skin.

Now, each and every day millions of dead skin cells are being sloughed away. (In fact, every month or so, you have a completely new epidermis. A whole new superficial you!) So as your old epidermis wears off, so does your sunless tan. That's why self-tanners have to be reapplied every few days to maintain the maximum effect.

So if you covet that rich year-round tan, here are your choices: You can move to Florida or Southern California and slather yourself with baby oil and sit out on your patio all day with one of those aluminum reflectors—although you'll be seriously courting melanoma (and at the very least probably end up looking like all my grandmother's leathery friends who used to sit outside their swim-club cabanas in the sun, the reptilian flab dangling from their upper arms as they shuffled their mah-jongg tiles). Or you can routinely rotisserie yourself in a tanning booth, which also poses some potential UV overexposure risk. Or you can take a tanning pill, most of which contain something called canthaxanthin, which is NOT approved by the FDA for use as a tanning agent, and which will not only turn your skin a nice Oompa-Loompa orange, but will also tint your tears, sweat, pee, and poop, AND which has been linked to hepatitis and something called canthaxanthin retinopathy (a condition in which yellow deposits form in the retina of your eye).

So you might just want to coat your bad self with that self-tanner … Just remember to rebaste every few weeks after molting.

Can you get toe fungus from a pedicure?

Is there danger lurking down at the local nail salon? The fungus among us is something doctors affectionately call onychomycosis, and it's fairly common. Some 15 percent of us have it and almost half of people over the age of seventy suffer from this ailment, which causes the toenail—particularly on the big toe—to become thick and discolored. Toenails are a cozy environment for the fungus because they are usually dark and damp, and dark and damp is heaven for fungi.

Toenail fungus can sometimes get better on its own, but usually worsens without treatment. Prescription medication used to treat toenail fungus includes fluconazole (Diflucan), and terbinafine (Lamisil). Onychomycosis is contagious and, yes, you can get it at a nail salon.

But you can also get it in a shower stall, a locker room, a bathroom, or from sharing a nail file or emery board with a friend or family member who has toe fungus. So, please don't deprive yourself of the pleasure of a pedicure, just be careful.

If you want to pamper your little piggies at a salon, make sure that it has a current operating license, and that its instruments are properly sanitized. Autoclaving (heat sterilization) of the instruments is best, but germicidal chemical sterilization will also suffice. You can also always bring your own set of toe tools.

Can you get herpes from a hot tub?

So, you settle in for a nice soak, without a care in the world. But is there danger lurking in the water?

Well, we don't want to be the bearers of bad news, but if that whirlpool or hot tub isn't properly cleaned or chlorinated, you could end up with a nice body rash. The Centers for Disease Control and Prevention (CDC) reported in 2004 that "Extensive spa use combined with inadequate maintenance contribute to recreational water illnesses (RWIs) caused by pathogens such as pseudomonas spp., legionella spp., and mycobacterium spp." Yuck.

It's not as bad as it sounds. Pseudomonas folliculitis (hot-tub folliculitis) is a skin infection that can develop within forty-eight hours after a dip in the spa. It is caused by bacteria getting into the hair follicles. You then get red, round, itchy bumps that later can develop into small pus-filled blisters. The rash usually resolves spontaneously within two to ten days.

As for the herpes question, the chlorine in hot tubs should kill the herpes virus. There are reports of people catching herpes skin infections from hot tubs, but these are very rare.

Why does your skin get thinner as you age?

As we get older, there are some unavoidable process-es at work that age our skin. This is something we will all experience and there's not really much we can do to prevent it. When a person ages, his or her epider-mal cells—the cells at the outer skin layer—become thinner, which makes the skin appear noticeably thin-ner. And the number of pigment-containing cells called melanocytes decrease, which can make your skin look more pale and translucent. Also, less colla-gen is produced, causing something called elastosis, which results in a reduction of the skin's strength and elasticity, and sagging and wrinkles. Then there's also a lifetime of exposure to the sun's ultraviolet radiation to be factored in … Not an especially glamorous pic-ture, I suppose. But, hey, it sure beats the alternative.

Anyway, don't worry. As old as you get, you will never become completely transparent so people can see your internal organs and skeleton.

Yes, I had one of those transparent anatomical dolls when I was a kid, and I had a G.I. Joe too. So?

Chapter 9

Growing Pains: FAQs About Puberty and Kids

A rejuvenated Leyner, back from his extended vacation in Upstate New York, was ready to return to patient care.

I had tried to keep our practice limited to individual therapy and couples' counseling. I had some trepidation that exposing a vulnerable adolescent mind to Leyner's disturbing therapeutic modalities would be very dangerous. Unfortunately, we had to make an exception when one of our couples insisted upon bringing their fourteen-year-old daughter in for a session.

I had known Ralph and Cindy Tucker for several years prior to working with Leyner. Ralph was an insurance agent who specialized in physician disability and malpractice insurance. His wife was the office manager and an accomplished horticulturalist. Leyner and I had worked with them during a difficult period when Cindy and Ralph were briefly separated. We were particularly touched last Christmas when we received a box of Cindy's prized tulip bulbs and a school photograph of their thirteen-year-old daughter, Stacey, a beaming little girl with pigtails and braces.

Ralph and Cindy entered our office accompanying what I can only describe as the spitting image of Anna Kournikova—a beautiful blond, lithe, and curvaceous young woman, her long hair flowing down to the small of her back. She was wearing a T-shirt that read "Squeeze Me, I'm Juicy."

I was a little confused. "Ralph, Cindy—I thought you were bringing your daughter today?"

"We did. Stacey, this is Dr. Goldberg and that's Leyner."

The poised young woman shook our hands. "It's a pleasure meeting you both. I was just curious—who wrote 'sniff my crotch' on the Van Gogh outside?"

I looked over at Leyner, expecting one of his pre-dictably inappropriate responses.

Leyner shifted in his seat and responded, "Oh, a particularly deranged individual did that. We decided to leave it."

"I'm glad you did," she said. "It's very refreshing."

I thought we should begin the session. I asked Ralph and Cindy exactly why they had come to see us today. They looked at each other lovingly but concerned, and Ralph began to answer.

"I um … we uhh …" he stammered. Cindy saw he was floundering and stepped in. "We think that Stacey will be reaching puberty soon and we thought it would be helpful to discuss some of the changes she might expect with professionals."

I couldn't look at Leyner. He remained silent.

I glanced over at Stacey. She rolled her eyes and stared at her parents with a surprising lack of judgment and a precocious sense of loving empathy and indulgence.

"Ralph, do you agree with what Cindy said?" I asked.

"Umm, uhhhh, yeah," he responded.

I didn't know quite how to phrase this delicately, so I decided to be somewhat blunt: "Sometimes it's difficult for a parent to perceive changing facets within an otherwise inherently familiar domestic environment in the context of rapid and tectonic hormonal changes and libidinal contradictions especially when it's exacerbated by a repressed albeit nostalgic tendency to embrace an idealized past."

Leyner laughed and couldn't help himself. "I'd concur if I had the slightest idea what you just said."

Stacey jumped right in. "I think what Dr. Goldberg was attempting to say is that my parents are having a hard time coming to terms with the fact that I had my period, I have boobs, and I think a lot about sex."

There was a long, long silence that permeated the room.

Ralph had turned a bizarre shade of red, Cindy was fidgeting uncontrollably, but Leyner remained remarkably calm.

I looked at my watch and wondered what I could possibly say to fill the remaining forty-three minutes.

Leyner stood up. I braced myself for the worst.

He cleared his throat and said, "I can only marvel at the grace and wisdom of your daughter. You should be very proud of her. Let's pick up here next week."

The Tucker family seemed relieved that the session was over.

Leyner escorted the three from the office, and upon returning, promptly collapsed in a heap on the floor.

Obviously the enormous effort at self-control and decorum had completely exhausted him, and we were forced to cancel the remaining patients for the day.

Why is one of my breasts growing faster than the other?

None of us is perfectly symmetrical. Unfortunately, especially for girls growing up in our culture, we spend an inordinate amount of time emulating the seemingly perfect bisymmetry of people like Jessica Simpson, Tyra Banks, and, of course, Barbie. But unless you're made out of extruded plastic in a mold in some factory in Malaysia, there are probably slight variances between one side of yourself and the other, whether it's your ears, big toes, or even breasts. And this is especially true when your body is developing during puberty.

The development of breast "buds" (small mounds beneath the nipple and areola) is usually the first sign of the onset of puberty in girls. As your body begins producing higher levels of female hormones, your breasts will go through five "stages" of growth. It is not uncommon for one breast to start growing before the other (sometimes even six months apart) and many girls' breasts develop unevenly. But this is perfectly normal. And the difference in breast size usually decreases as your breasts develop. Your breasts will reach full maturity by the age of seventeen or eighteen, and their final size is determined by heredity.

Instead of becoming self-conscious and getting all freaked out about things other people probably don't even notice, you might try ridiculing the bodies of famous people. Making fun of the physical imperfections of celebrities is not only a constructive and enjoyable way to sublimate your own body dysmorphia, but it's the new national pastime.

Do growing pains really exist?

Growing up—in and of itself—is an enormous pain in the butt. The grades, the melodramatic infatuations, the looming necessity of earning a living … And hey, why do homework when, in 5 billion years, the sun is going to exhaust all its nuclear fuel and collapse into a dead, cold, shrunken cinder? And I didn't ask to be born anyway … Oh, sorry—I'm getting a little carried away with all the adolescent angst …

What about those folkloric "growing pains"? There is no evidence that growing—the normal development of bones and joints and muscles—causes any pain. But many parents have experienced their children waking up in the middle of the night and complaining, for example, that their legs are sore. And because their children are in the midst of a growth spurt, the growth and the discomfort seem to be somehow connected. But this is not the case. Most probably your child has had a particularly active or strenuous or rough-and-tumble day of running and jumping and climbing, and all this activity can be tough on a kid's joints and muscles. What he or she probably needs is some tender reassurance and perhaps a nice massage and some good ol'-fashioned cuddling. In the morning, the wee one should be fit as a fiddle. (If you think there's been some injury, or if there's persistent pain, or his or her joints are tender to the touch, or there's a fever or a rash, your child should be taken to a doctor for an examination.)

Being awakened late at night by a child complaining of vague aches and pains can be annoying. But try to be patient. It probably won't help much to accuse your child of "faking" symptoms for attention or to get out of going to school the next day.

By the way, when it comes to faking illness to get out of going to school (or "juvenile malingering"), Leyner could write the authoritative how-to guide. In an effort to evade the indignities of first grade, he perfected the art of using the hot bulb of his night-table lamp to heat a thermometer to a perfect 101 degrees—not too high a fever, but just enough to miss school. (This ruse requires an extremely adroit technique to prevent registering a shockingly high temperature that results in a day spent in the ER and not lounging around the house in pajamas with your mom waiting on you hand and foot.) Leyner was also skilled in convincingly simulating an exotic array of early-morning symptoms (for example, cyanosis, torticollis, and rectal prolapse) that makes Ferris Bueller look like a rank amateur.

Why can kids tolerate cold pool or ocean water better than adults?

It's a classic scene. The shivering kid with the blue lips and chattering teeth, who vehemently denies that he's cold and refuses to get out of the pool or come to shore. Does this mean that children are somehow more capable of enduring cold temperatures than adults? No. What it means is that children will universally resist any suggestion that they stop doing something fun. It means that children are acutely susceptible to peer pressure. It means that children take great, perverse pleasure in disobeying and alarming their parents. But it does not mean that they are less vulnerable to the cold. On the contrary, children are more susceptible to hypothermia and frostbite than adults. Kids cool faster than adults. And, due to a variety of factors—including size, heat generation, and vasomotor control—they are less able to thermoregulate in the cold. So when your kid is inebriated on sheer glee and seems oblivious to frigid temperatures, exercising some caution is actually a very good idea.

What is a wet dream?

A wet dream, otherwise known as a "nocturnal emission," is the involuntary ejaculation of semen from the penis during sleep—an orgasm while you doze. They are most common when boys enter puberty and during the teenage years, but they can occur at any time during a man's life. They are, like, totally normal. Many boys experience spontaneous erections during sleep. Nocturnal emissions can be the result of sexual excitement from erotic dreams, or physical stimulation from rubbing against sheets or blankets, etc. Sometimes you might wake up during a wet dream, but frequently you sleep right through it. So a wet dream might very well be a guy's first experience of not only falling asleep after sex, but of actually sleeping during sex.

Dreams are wonderful things. In dreams, we can have sex with Academy Award-winning actresses, porn stars, reality TV personalities, neighbors, coworkers, teachers, girls who ignored us in high school, our friends' moms, babysitters from childhood, that waitress from the German restaurant, cartoon characters … (What? You don't think Smurfette is hot?)

And sometimes the dream can have a real Happy Ending.

3:33 p.m.
Gberg: Professor Leyner? Are you at the research institute?

3:35 p.m.
Leyner: I was researching the exciting

tragicomic world of nocturnal emissions.

Gberg: I just read that Grandpa Munster died.

Leyner: NO!?

Gberg: Not sure what the nocturnal emission connection is.

Gberg: He was 95.

Leyner: Maybe he died of a nocturnal emission. It can happen.

Gberg: Cum and go at the same time.

Leyner: You can aspirate your own jizz ... and die.

Gberg: It says his wife was at the bedside. You never know.

Gberg: Are you still obsessed with that book you are reading?

Leyner: Speaking of cumming and going ... did you hear that Lance Armstrong and Sheryl Crowe are finished?? (Yes, I'm more obsessed than ever with Lord Nelson ... I feel a great affinity with him.)

Gberg: Affinity for Lance Armstrong or Lord Nelson?

Leyner: Lord Nelson ... c'mon.

3:40 p.m.

Gberg: On the nocturnal-emission front, I found an article about sleep sex, sex while sleepwalking.

Gberg: Has a Leyneresque ring to it.

Leyner: Sex while sleeping ... that's terrific.

Leyner: I love that idea ... you're asleep ... you get up ... start wandering around ...

Gberg: From the *Archives of Sexual Behavior*.

Gberg: I love the names of some of these journals, they sound made up.

Leyner: Arms extended in front of you ... in classic somnambulant pose.

Gberg: I just quoted the *Journal of Chemical Senses*.

Leyner: And then ... you use your little plastic hotel key-card and get into some business-woman's room—she's on some trip promoting her company's new exfoliant or something—AND ... you get in ...

Leyner: There's a *Journal of Chemical Senses*?

Gberg: Yes, and don't joke about the sleep sex, they describe a case of sexual battery where they use "somnambulism" as a defense.

Gberg: There also is sleep eating.

Leyner: And you slide into bed with her ... in your sleep, right? And ever so gently penetrate her as she dreams of huge puffins and pirates.

3:45 p.m.

Gberg: You are a sick man. Lord Nelson would be so proud!

Leyner: And in the a.m., no one's the worse for wear, because what happens in Jersey City, stays in Jersey City.

Leyner: If a person can run a country for eight

years, simpering and drooling and obviously
asleep—surely somnambulant sex is possible.

Gberg: He was asleep when he gave the state of
the union last week.

Why do boys sleep later in the morning during puberty?

Life requires at least three ingredients—water, heat,
and carbon-based molecules. With adolescents,
there's a fourth requirement: beds.

Almost all teens—male and female—seem to
crave the opportunity to "sleep in." This probably
seems more pronounced in boys, because it doesn't
seem so long ago when your little tyke was up at the
crack of dawn—maddeningly early—chomping at
the bit to play or build a treehouse or go ice-fishing
or shoot quail, any of those all-American things little
boys want to do at ungodly hours when normal
human beings just want to sleep. Then they hit
puberty.

Before puberty, kids' bodies signal that they are
sleepy at about 8 or 9 p.m. With the onset of puberty,
kids don't start feeling sleepy until around 10 or 11
p.m. This shift in an adolescent's circadian rhythms
(the body's twenty-four-hour cycles) is called "sleep-
phase delay"—a tendency toward later times for
both falling asleep and waking up.

Melatonin is a hormone made by a part of the brain called the pineal gland. It is thought to help our bodies know when it's time to go to sleep and when it's time to wake up. An experiment conducted at Brown University showed that melatonin secretion occurs at a later time in adolescents as they mature. It also showed that melatonin secretion turned off later in the morning, making it more difficult to wake up early.

Why do boys' breasts grow during puberty?

I guess you're never too young to begin worrying about the dreaded "man-boobs." Plus, there'd be no summer-camp comedies at the multiplex, unless bullies were able to mercilessly torment some poor, lovable soul with a conspicuous cup size.

When those hormones produced in the testicles to fuel puberty begin kicking in, many boys will develop some breast tissue. And this slight swelling under the nipples may persist for several years. But don't worry. This is perfectly normal and it certainly doesn't mean that you're growing breasts. About 65 percent of boys will develop some breast tissue—so it's very common and very temporary. Unless you have a serious weight problem, this breast tissue should be all gone by the time you are twenty.

Why does your voice change at puberty?

Ah, yes, what a dignified time of life—when, in the course of the same sentence, you can sound like Arnold Schwarzenegger and Alvin the Chipmunk.

Your larynx is a hollow, tube-shaped piece of cartilage that is located at the top of your trachea (windpipe). There are two thin muscles—called vocal cords—that are stretched across the trachea, sort of like rubber bands. And when you speak or sing, air rushing from your lungs causes these vocal cords to vibrate, producing your voice.

During puberty, higher levels of testosterone cause the cartilage of a boy's larynx to grow and the vocal cords to become longer and thicker, vibrating at a lower frequency, and creating a deeper tone of voice. There are other anatomical changes that contribute to the differences in an adolescent boy's voice. His facial bones begin to grow, as do his sinus cavities, nose, and throat. This creates a larger space in which his voice can resonate more deeply. (Some of this is actually visible—as the larynx gets bigger, it also tilts at a different angle and protrudes farther. Yes, boys and girls—the Adam's apple.)

That cracking and breaking voice that can mortify a pubescent boy is simply the result of his body adjusting to all of these physical changes. This is all very temporary. Once maturity and full laryngeal growth are achieved, those unpredictable squeaks become a thing of the past.

Does drinking milk really make you taller?

We know our response to this one is going to be greeted with howls of indignant protest from moms all over the world … But the answer is no.

There is no special "growth factor" in milk. Not that milk and other calcium-rich dairy products aren't wonderfully nutritious. Calcium is essential for helping promote stronger bones. And if you don't get a sufficient amount of calcium in your diet, your body compensates and basically steals it from your bones. This can eventually lead to osteoporosis—a steady, progressive loss of bone density that can cause people to become hunched over as they get older.

Height is the result of a complicated assortment of genetic factors and environmental interactions. It is polygenic—which means that many genes are involved. This is why sometimes children are significantly different heights than their parents. (The legendary basketball player and sex machine Wilt Chamberlain was 7 feet 1 inch. But neither of his parents rose above 5 feet 9 inches.) And height is multifactorial. In addition to the complex genetic component, many lifestyle factors—especially the mother's diet and health while she is pregnant and the nutrition of the child during the growth years—determine whether a person will attain his or her potential genetic height.

FYI—within the last hundred years or so, the Dutch have gone from being the shortest people in Europe to the tallest in the world. The average Dutch man today is 6 feet 1 inch. The average American man is only 5 feet 9½ inches.

Height is a critically important subject for Leyner. Although he ultimately achieved the imposing stature of 5 feet 7 inches, he was a shrimp of a kid. In an autobiographical account he wrote recently for *Best Life* magazine, he explains that his adult obsession with weight lifting "was a long overdue response to the cumulative traumas of having been picked on as a small boy. My parents doted on me as if I were some delicate, Proustian genius prince, but once I left the cultured confines of my own home, it was *Lord of the Flies* out there. As my father's career as an attorney flourished, we moved frequently, and every first day at a new school presented a new gauntlet of bullies … " Leyner goes on to describe the following shocking scene:

We'd just moved from Jersey City to West Orange, a seemingly benign middle-class bedroom community in the Jersey suburbs. One afternoon, on the way home from school, I'd followed a squirrel into the woods. (As an itinerant child who was typically friendless, I often found great solace in the companionship of small helpless creatures.)

There I was with my fey blond bangs and huge sparkly eyes, and as I tried to lure the squirrel closer with a tiny marzipan banana that my mother had packed as a surprise in my lunch that day, I was set upon by a pack of boys in blue uniforms. Crazed, sadistic Cub Scouts. It was like a scene from one of those Japanese schoolboy splatter films

Why do we have pubic hair?

This is a great conversation starter, if you're sitting on a plane or in line at the DMV … And it's not only the why, it's the where. Why there? Why have human beings been left with tufts of hair surrounding our genitals and in our armpits?

This isn't the place for a debate about evolution versus intelligent design, but pubic hair might seem to indicate a Creator with a very frat-boy sense of humor.

If you accost random people on the street and ask them why they have pubic hair, one of three things will happen: 1. They'll call a cop. 2. They shrug and guess, "To keep my, uh, private parts warm … ?" 3. They stiffen their posture, look you directly in the eye, and assert, "To protect my genitals."

If the purpose of pubic hair was to keep our "private parts" nice and toasty, wouldn't we have more of it and wouldn't it be much thicker? And if we depended on hair for warmth at this point in our evolution, wouldn't we be covered with fur?

As for protection, even so eminent an evolution-ary biologist as Mel Brooks has mused upon why the genitals—given their importance and sensitivity—are not encased in a small skull. And if pubic hair actually provided protection, wouldn't NFL players and racing-car drivers wear big bouffant wigs woven out of the short-and-curlies?

The most convincing hypothesis is that pubic hair—like axillary (armpit) hair—traps pheromones, those erotic scents that play such an important and fascinating role in human sexual communication. These pheromones are produced when the apocrine sweat glands release a viscous and odorless secretion on the skin surface that, when broken down by bac-teria, results in a characteristic sexual scent. Pubic hair and underarm hair are a human being's primary "scent traps." Mammalian pheromones influence the secretion of gonadotropin-releasing hormone (GnRH), a hormone that has short- and long-term effects on neurotransmission. Studies (including vari-ous smelly T-shirt-sniffing experiments) have shown that human pheromones have a significant effect on the attractiveness of one sex to the other.

Odor is such a crucial component of mammalian mating. With all the deodorants, colognes, douches, and Brazilian waxes out there—it's a wonder anyone can find a date anymore.

Does falling in love really cause chemical changes in your brain?

Why does falling in love turn seemingly rational, even-keeled, considerate people into deranged, raving, volatile, self-centered psychos in dire need of an exorcism, especially teenagers?

Welcome to Cupid's laboratory. There is indeed a biochemistry of love. Helen Fisher, an anthropology professor at Rutgers University—along with two colleagues, Arthur Aron and Lucy Brown—used an MRI machine to study the brains of people who describe themselves as being wildly "in love." When each subject gazed at a photograph of his or her sweetheart, the ventral tegmental area and the caudate nucleus lit up. The caudate nucleus is the site of a dense network of receptors for the neurotransmitter dopamine. Donatella Marazziti, a psychiatry professor at the University of Pisa in Italy, measured the serotonin levels of the neurotransmitter serotonin in the blood of people who'd been in love for several months and who pine or are otherwise preoccupied with their lovers for at least four hours a day. She found that the serotonin levels in the love-struck subjects were as low as the serotonin levels in people with obsessive-compulsive disorder (OCD).

So if you're feeling "madly" in love, or a little "insane in the membrane," or "crazy, crazy for feeling so lonely," there's a solid, scientific basis for losing your heart AND your marbles.

Does television really rot kids' brains?

How many parents have gazed despairingly at their children who sit comatose in front of the TV for what seems like eons of uninterrupted viewing, their eyes glazed, their sallow faces awash in that bluish glow? Surely this is rotting their brains, wiping clean whole neural networks, all cognitive functioning flickering off, neuron by neuron and synapse by synapse with each ensuing episode of *American Idol*, *The Apprentice*, *Survivor*, and *The Biggest Loser*. And instead of high-functioning, productive members of society of whom they can be justifiably proud, parents fear being saddled with zombies in hairnets, muttering, "You want fries with that?" for the rest of their lives. And it's all the TV's fault, right?

Wrong. A new study by two economists from the University of Chicago, Matthew Gentzkow and Jesse M. Shapiro, shows "very little difference and if anything, a slight positive advantage" in test scores for kids who grew up watching TV early on, as compared to kids who did not. And in households where English was a second language or the mom had less than a high-school education, the positive effect of TV was even more pronounced. (This study was released by the National Bureau of Economic Research, a nonprofit, nonpartisan group of academic researchers in Cambridge, Massachusetts.)

New research also appears to debunk the notion

that TV shortens children's attention spans. A study recently published in the journal *Pediatrics* and based on American kindergartners, and another conducted in the Netherlands, found absolutely no link between television viewing and symptoms of attention-deficit disorder.

So, c'mon, kids! We apologize. Put those silly books down and come grab a seat in front of the 65-inch plasma … *The Simple Life* is on!!

Chapter 10

Natural and Unnatural Cures That We Want You to Know About

L eyner and I had a busy morning of patients and an intriguing mix of cases. Our last patient was a TV-obsessed housewife who spent her entire family's savings on products hawked on an endless variety of infomercials. She finally came to us when the last book she purchased failed to cure her depression, insomnia, and obsessive hypochondriasis. After a long session, I tried to engage Leyner in a discussion of the overwhelming susceptibility of people to untested cures and hyperbole. Leyner resisted and focused all of his energies on his more entrepreneurial side. I decided to take a break from the office and go for a solo lunch to ponder things.

When I returned from lunch, I found Leyner seated behind a desk with a bizarre miscellany of ingredients that he had purchased in Chinatown along with a Bunsen burner and mortar and pestle. Leyner was formulating some sort of exotic concoction made out of ground deer antler, desiccated seahorse, minced bear gallbladder, Siberian ginseng extract, and distilled ylang-ylang. Wendy was stationed behind a large tripod with a video camera aimed at Leyner's science experiment. Leyner carefully measured out several teaspoons of omega-3 fish oil and equal amounts of manganese and riboflavin. Using a pipette, he drew 10 milliliters of kiwi-strawberry Propel from a bottle and meticulously added it to the potion. "*Voilà!*" he pronounced proudly. He gave Wendy a signal to start shooting.

"And ... action!" she shouted.

"Hi there. I'm Mark Leyner. What you're about to hear will change not only your life, but the lives of those you love, and may very well alter the future of mankind itself. There are many organizations out there, which for their own selfish and nefarious reasons, don't want you to hear what I'm about to say ... the FDA, the AMA, the FCC, the FTC, the SEC, the AFL-CIO, the CIA, the NBA, and the PTA. But as an author and a healer, it is my responsibility to suffer the slings and arrows of the skeptics and naysayers in order to make this miraculous new product available to you as soon as possible.

"MegaProfen-10™ is a revolutionary supplement that can almost instantly transform you into a happy, vital human being with boundless energy and natural immunity to all the world's most devastating diseases and debilitating conditions. It has also been proven to add decades to your life span and imbue you with a radiant, indefatigable sexuality."

Leyner whispered to Wendy, "Go tight on me."

For his close-up, Leyner furrowed with great telegenic earnestness and concern.

"Are you suffering from sudden back spasms? Do night-time leg cramps keep you awake? Do you want to stop the embarrassment of diarrhea, gas, bloating, constipation, cramps, and incontinence, and regain the freedom of an active lifestyle? Do you want to slim down ugly bulges? Is your appearance marred by sagging skin, wrinkles, and unattractive 'turkey neck'? Is your libido faltering? Are you falling behind in school or job advancement because of limited intelligence? Do you have eczema or nail fungus? Do you have high cholesterol, acid reflux, Marburg hemorrhagic fever, or bovine spongiform encephalopathy? Well, it's time to stop worrying and reach for this little bottle—"

Leyner holds up the bottle and grins with great satisfaction, his teeth gleaming.

I couldn't hold back and had to interrupt. "Leyner, we're trying to be professionals and you can't go on TV and make ridiculous unfounded claims. Are you trying to ruin my reputation? Do you want to sabotage our practice?" I was fuming.

Leyner countered, "This country was founded on ridiculous unfounded claims. When Paul Revere said, 'The British are coming,' do you think there was incontrovertible proof? We're a nation of snake oil-quaffing pet rock owners and copper bracelet-wearing magnet worshippers. And I'm proud to be an American!"

"Wendy, did you get that?" Leyner asked.

I couldn't believe he was trying to drag me into this.

"You do not have my permission to include me in your charade!" I screamed as I went into my office and slammed the door.

Leyner waited a brief second and motioned to Wendy to roll the camera.

He settled himself, sat down, and reassumed his salesman-like demeanor of jaunty credibility.

"MegaProfen-10™ has been exhaustively tested in our state-of-the-art laboratories and received the full and unequivocal endorsement of … Dr. Billy Goldberg."

Why should you breathe into a paper bag when hyperventilating?

This is a classic home remedy and something that we occasionally rely on in the emergency room, but not everyone who is hyperventilating should be given the bag. Hyperventilation is a fancy word for rapid deep breathing. It is usually caused by anxiety or panic, but many conditions can cause hyperventilation including: asthma, heart attack, bleeding, pneumonia, overdoses, and stimulant use. In patients with heart attacks, collapsed lungs, or blood clots in the lungs death can occur if they are misdiagnosed and treated with paper-bag rebreathing. Once we decide that you don't have something serious, we will reach for the bag. So let your doctor make this diagnosis!

Breathing into a paper bag works by making you rebreathe the carbon dioxide that you are exhaling. This causes the blood levels of carbon dioxide to rise, and slows your breathing.

Instead of using the bag, you can slow your breathing by breathing through pursed lips or by breathing from the diaphragm. If you do reach for the bag, know that there is no magic chemical in the brown paper bag, and you probably could use your empty McDonald's bag or even your Prada purse.

Do those instant hand sanitizers really work?

Does washing your hands really prevent disease?

The answer is a resounding yes! Few things are as certain as this in medicine. There is no doubt that washing your hands can prevent disease.

The problem is getting people to do it. A study in the *Annals of Internal Medicine* looked at the rate of hand-washing among physicians and found that doctors washed their hands only 57 percent of the time they should have. This is higher than many studies that have shown compliance rates lower than 50 percent. In this study, the adherence to hand hygiene rates varied by specialty with internal medicine doctors washing the most, and anesthesiologists the least. Medical students did better than their professors, and female physicians did better than their male counterparts. The presence of a hand-rub solution increased the compliance with hand-washing.

For this reason, those alcohol-based hand-rub solutions are all over hospitals. The good news is that they work well too. The CDC in their *Guideline for Hand Hygiene in Health-Care Settings* state that "Alcohol-based products are more effective for standard hand-washing or hand antisepsis by health-care workers than soap or antimicrobial soap." But these hand rubs are not appropriate for use when hands are visibly soiled or after going to the bathroom.

As for the omnipresence of antibacterial soap, it is

not necessary. The most important thing is to rub your hands vigorously together while washing and continue for ten to fifteen seconds. The regular soap and the scrubbing action together will help wash away the germs.

Do copper bracelets help with rheumatism?

This was a question from Billy's wife's grandmother. We love the term "rheumatism." It's so old-fashioned and dramatic and makes you think about other illnesses like lumbago, dropsy, or the fits. Rheumatism isn't a term that is used in hospitals, but is generally used to refer to arthritis.

Arthritis doesn't refer to one specific condition, but is a general term for inflammation of the joints. There are over one hundred types of arthritis, and it affects about 42 million people. The most common form of arthritis is osteoarthritis. Osteoarthritis is caused by wear and tear on the joints and ultimately the breakdown and loss of cartilage. There is no cure for osteoarthritis.

Copper bracelets have been sold as a cure for arthritis based upon the belief that the copper is absorbed into the skin and can help rejuvenate the cartilage. This is a myth, and there is no proof that these bracelets work. There are many studies looking at copper and how it affects the growth of cartilage, so in the future we may discover some new ways to use this important element. Copper is, however, a necessary part of our diet. Copper is essential for normal metabolism, but copper deficiency is extremely uncommon. In the meantime, there are serious side effects with copper supplements. So check with your doctor before taking them.

As for the copper bracelets, go ahead, wear them if you want. They won't fix your arthritis, but they might turn your arm green.

Can you get the flu from a flu shot?

Influenza (the flu) is different from the common cold. Both are caused by viruses and can produce the same symptoms, but the flu is generally much more severe. Most people describe higher temperatures and severe body aches when they have the flu and not a cold.

A flu vaccine contains inactivated viruses (viruses that are killed), so you cannot get the flu from a flu shot. The shot is designed to allow your body to develop protection (antibodies) without actually getting sick. This happens about two weeks after receiving the vaccine. Up to that point, you are still at risk of getting the flu, just not from the shot.

Minor side effects associated with the flu vaccine include soreness, redness, or swelling at the injection site, low-grade fever, and body aches. The flu vaccine doesn't provide 100 percent protection against getting the flu. Experts try to predict the strain for that year, and match the vaccine with the virus. As you probably know by now, experts aren't always right.

Is it true that laughter has healing powers?

So, you are now on page 235 of this book. C'mon, tell us you're not feeling a little better.

You might be surprised to know that there is significant evidence that humor can do a body good. Perhaps you have read "Modulation of Neuroimmune Parameters During the Eustress of Humor-associated Mirthful Laughter" in the March 2001 issue of *Alternative Therapies in Health & Medicine*. This study tested blood samples of over fifty men, before and after they viewed a one-hour humor video.

Scientists measured some hilarious things like "Natural-killer-cell activity, plasma immunoglobulins, B cells, T cells with helper and suppressor markers, total leukocytes with subpopulations of lymphocytes, granulocytes, and monocytes, etc." They found increases in many of these cells, which suggests a link between humor, laughter, and positive health benefits. Now, this isn't incontrovertible science, but there certainly aren't any unpleasant side effects of laughter.

For the more pious among us, an even earlier allusion to a link between laughter and health can be found in the Bible: "A merry heart doeth good like a medicine" (*Proverbs* 17:22).

Why can we still not cure the common cold?

We can map the human genome, clone a sheep, send a man to the moon, and even infuse bottled water with 100 percent of the daily recommended allowance of vitamins and minerals … So how is it that we still can't cure the common cold?

It's not as though scientists haven't tried. It's just that the odds are stacked against them. To begin with, at least two hundred identified viruses are capable of causing the collection of symptoms that we identify as a cold. These viruses include rhino viruses, coronaviruses, parainfluenza viruses, respiratory syncytial virus, adenoviruses, and enteroviruses. Rhinoviruses are responsible for about 70 percent of all infections, but even among the rhinoviruses, there are many different types. Another trouble with these viruses is that they keep mutating. This makes finding a cure almost impossible.

The best hope lies with a vaccine, but with around two hundred viruses that change every year, we would probably need just as many shots on a yearly basis to prevent colds. Maybe it's better to just take some anti-inflammatories and cuddle up on the couch with a box of tissues, some chicken soup, and the remote control.

Why don't people who take nitroglycerin for their heart ever blow up?

If you are a fan of the old Roadrunner cartoons, you probably remember the coyote blowing himself up time and time again trying to handle explosive nitroglycerin. If the coyote had so many troubles, why can heart patients carry around their nitroglycerin pills without any danger?

This question is made even more intriguing by the fact that there is no chemical difference between the nitroglycerin used in explosives and in heart medication.

For those who don't know what nitroglycerin or "nitro" is, it is a medication used for the prevention and treatment of heart attacks. Nitroglycerin comes in tablets, ointment, patches, sprays, and most commonly a small pill that is placed under the tongue. Nitroglycerin dilates (opens) blood vessels, increasing blood flow to areas of the heart that are being deprived of oxygen.

A good way to understand why therapeutic nitro doesn't blow up is to consider dynamite. Dynamite, which is safe to handle, also contains nitroglycerin. In dynamite, the nitroglycerin is combined (or diluted) with a nonexplosive substance, diatomaceous earth. Dynamite is then stable enough to handle and resists shocks and movement. All you need is a blasting cap and you are ready to blow stuff up.

The medicinal dose of nitroglycerin is infinitesimal compared with the amount in a stick of dynamite. So kids out there—don't try to steal your father's nitro, attach a blasting cap, and blow up the neighbor's cat.

When you use products for hair loss, does hair just grow on your head or on your whole body?

There are many options for people who are suffering from hair loss. Options include shaving it all off like Kojak or Michael Jordan, growing the remaining hair as long as possible and attempting a "comb-over," or taking the toupee route. If none of these choices work for you, there are medications that can stimulate hair growth.

Minoxidil (Rogaine) and finasteride (Propecia) are the two best-known medications to try to regain that shaggy look. Minoxidil was a drug originally used to treat high blood pressure, that is, until it was found to increase body hair growth. This side effect led to the development of a topical solution that could be applied directly to the scalp. The exact mechanism of action of minoxidil is unknown, but somehow it stimulates the follicles to create new hairs. The treatment must be continued indefinitely in order to maintain hair growth, because we keep getting new hair follicles and we need to continue exposing them to the medication.

Although minoxidil is a topical treatment, some of the drug can be absorbed into your system, and unwanted body hair has been reported. If you are not careful when applying it and it gets onto other body parts, they can also get hairier.

Finasteride is a prescription drug that comes in tablet form to treat hair loss in men only. (Minoxidil works for men or women.) It was originally used for the treatment of prostate enlargement. Finasteride works by blocking an enzyme responsible for the conversion of testosterone to dihydrotestosterone (DHT). Men with male-pattern hair loss (androgenic alopecia) tend to have miniaturized hair follicles and increased amounts of DHT on their scalps compared with those with hairier heads. The reduction in the amount of DHT can help reverse the balding process and stimulate new hair growth. Results are usually seen in about three months. The specific enzyme that is blocked by this drug is only found in the prostate, the liver, and the scalp, so there shouldn't be any effect on hair on other parts of the body.

Does ginger have any medicinal qualities?

In the Goldberg and Leyner families, the first thing our mothers did when we had stomachaches was reach for ginger ale.

Ginger has been studied for a variety of medical purposes for many years. In China, it is often prescribed for headaches, stomach problems, and the common cold. Indian practitioners of aryuvedic medicine also use it for digestion and arthritis. In the West, it is used most commonly for the prevention of nausea.

There are many scientific studies about different uses of ginger, but the only use whose efficacy is clinically proven is for the treatment of nausea and vomiting associated with pregnancy. In low doses, ginger may be appropriate for pregnant patients, but check with your doctor first.

Despite the best intentions of our mothers, commercially available ginger ale doesn't even contain any real ginger. But it still seemed to work. That's the placebo effect. Thanks anyway, Mom.

Can garlic prevent heart disease or cancer?

Many common medications that doctors use come from natural sources. Warfarin, a common blood thinner, was discovered from bleeding cows that had eaten yellow sweet clover. Digitalis, a heart medication, is derived from the plant foxglove, and penicillin comes from the penicillium mold. Recent studies point to the antioxidant properties of red wine, pomegranate juice, and dark chocolate. And ethnobotanists are scouring the Amazon to explore the medicinal potential of indigenous flora. So what about garlic?

We love garlic, but unfortunately there just isn't any data in yet that decisively proves this pungent bulb's health benefits. Garlic has been studied in high blood pressure, cholesterol lowering, blood thinning, and cancer prevention, to name a few. The best available data suggest that garlic is slightly better than a placebo in reducing total cholesterol levels, but this effect is debatable.

Don't worry, when we find more evidence, we will let you know and we can all go out and celebrate by gorging ourselves on a huge plate of shrimps. Until then, feel free to wear a clove around your neck or hang it on your door to keep evil spirits and vampires at bay.

Do magnets work to cure pain?

Thanks to a variety of questionable claims, the medical magnet business is booming. Annual sales are about $300 million in the United States alone and over $1 billion worldwide. Magnets have been said to increase circulation, reduce inflammation, speed recovery from injuries, relieve low back pain, and even increase longevity and aid in cancer treatment. None of these claims are supported by any data.

There are two types of magnets: static (permanent) magnets whose electromagnetic fields are unchanging (these are the ones that are marketed to gullible grandmas) and electromagnets that generate magnetic fields only when electric current flows through them. In the future, science may find roles for the use of electromagnets, but we doubt that static magnets will ever have any utility.

One best-selling author, a vociferous proponent of magnet therapy, urges us to "neutralize electromagnetic chaos." How do you do that, you might ask? You run out and buy an Electromagnetic Chaos Eliminator Pendant, stupid. Feel free to waste your money if you wish.

We think a better use of magnets is for sticking your kids' artwork to the fridge.

Do doctors really still use maggots and leeches?

It's not uncommon for us to see a homeless patient come in with a leg infection that is covered in maggots. After we brush away the "bugs" (maggots are actually flies at a larval stage), the wounds are surprisingly clean.

Yes, maggots eat away dead tissue and leave only the healthy stuff behind. This is not a very appetizing solution, but it works, and doctors have indeed used these little creatures as a therapy for cleaning stubborn wounds. Sterile maggots of the green bottle fly, *Lucilia sericata*, are used for this procedure, which is called "maggot debridement therapy." The maggots (about five to ten) are placed on each square centimeter of a wound. The wound is then covered with a breathable protective dressing and the maggots are left for about two to three days to do their work. Not only do the maggots eat the infected tissue, it is believed that they secrete substances that kill bacteria and promote wound healing.

Now for the leeches ...

Medical leeches are making a comeback, but it's not for those good old bloodlettings. The use of leeches in medicine dates back to antiquity. The first use of a medical leech was about 1000 b.c., probably in ancient India. They reached their peak of popularity in the nineteenth century. Leeches were used for a variety of ailments, the idea being that blood carried evil humors and that thinning the blood would lead to good health. Leeching fell from favor, but today, the little bloodsuckers are used by plastic surgeons throughout the world as tools in skin grafts and reattachment surgery.

If you want to read an intriguing tale about medical leeches, get a copy of *The New Yorker* from July 25, 2005, and enjoy John Colapinto's article "Bloodsuckers." You can learn that "Leeches are found in virtually every kind of habitat—including a species in the Sahara that resides in the noses of camels; one that resides in the anuses of hippopotamuses; a cave-dwelling leech in New Guinea that sucks on the blood of bats; and one that attacks the armpits of turtles." The leech used for medical purposes doesn't come from a hippo anus, it is a European leech, *Hirudo medicinalis*, that is raised on leech farms.

Leeches do their work by removing blood from the site of skin grafts or reattached parts and relieving congestion in the blood vessels. The Hirudo leech also has a chemical in its saliva that acts as an anticoagulant to prevent blood clotting. The bite of a leech is painless due to its own anesthetic.

• Chapter 11 •

The Lost and Found Department: A Random Assortment of Questions

When I came into the office I found Leyner in the middle of the floor doing a rapid series of one-handed push-ups. He noticed my arrival, bounced up, and ran over to me with great excitement. If he had a tail, I am sure it would have been wagging.

"Man, today is going to be great! Last night I went to a lecture at NYU by the world-renowned group therapy guru Andrew Weissman. I figured out the best way to test his methods."

Leyner grabbed my arm and pulled me out of the office.

245

He led me around the corner to our favorite local bakery. The place was packed—there must have been at least a hundred people jammed in—and I saw Wendy stationed behind the counter. As we entered, I heard her shout, "Okay, everyone, we'll be starting soon. Does everybody have a number?" She pointed toward the classic red bakery ticket dispenser.

Leyner escorted me behind the counter and turned to me to explain his experiment. "I was thinking … seeing one patient every hour is stupid … we're totally limiting how much cash we can make. I went out last night after the lecture and found tons of people with a wide variety of illnesses who were looking for a quick fix. This is genius … it's like McTherapy."

"Leyner, you can't treat people with serious and complex psychological problems like fast-food customers. The human psyche is not a Big Mac."

"Who says? Wendy?"

"Number six?"

"Here!" Someone in the back shouted, waving his ticket in the air.

Leyner pointed at him. "What's your problem, sir? And try to keep it brief—we want to give everyone a chance."

The guy looked at Leyner and said, "I'm twenty-five, I still live with my parents, and I occasionally wet my bed. What can I do?"

Leyner didn't miss a beat. "Your bed-wetting is obviously due to the long-repressed traumas of toilet training. Move out, get rubber sheets, or sleep in a litter box. Next!"

"Number seven?"

"Yes," a weak tremulous female voice murmured from the left side of the room. "I … I'm … I've been very, very depressed since the death of my favorite aunt and I cry every time I see an older woman," she said, beginning to weep.

"Come on down!" Leyner shouted.

The woman shyly ambled to the counter. Leyner lay a hand on either shoulder and shook her violently.

"Out neurotic depression!" he bellowed. "I command you! OUT!!"

The woman crumpled to the ground, remained motionless for a second, and then sat up, grinning from ear to ear.

"Do you feel depressed anymore?" Leyner asked.

"No," replied the woman, looking around almost as if in disbelief. "I feel … happy! Thank you!!"

The crowd applauded.

"Wait," I said, and addressed the room. "Don't let Leyner force you to take part in this public spectacle. We all know there's no instant cure for childhood issues or depression. Therapy takes work and it takes time. There are many facilities across the city where—"

I was interrupted by a guy in the back who screamed out, "Hey, I got number sixteen and I gotta be back at work in a half hour. Stop your whining and let Leyner help us!"

"All right, then," Leyner beamed. "Number eight."

"Right here," announced a man in his mid-forties, wearing a polo shirt and jeans.

"Yes?" said Leyner, motioning for him to get on with it.

"I'm lonely. I've tried everything I know to meet someone … the bar scene, blind dates, online dating, matchmakers. Nothing's worked. I'm beginning to wonder if I'm just fated to spend the rest of my life alone."

The crowd audibly sighed.

"Your problem is you need a woman, right?" Leyner grabbed Wendy, and pushed her into the guy's arms. "Here you go. This is Wendy. Have fun. Number nine."

And so it went. I was amazed at the miscellaneous collection of desperate individuals that Leyner had assembled and how succinctly and peremptorily he satisfied their varied questions.

"Number twenty-eight. Number twenty-eight. Okay, twenty-nine."

A thin woman stepped forward and said, "Can I have one apple tart, two chocolate croissants, and …"

Leyner cut her off. "Aaah, obviously you're acting out a deep-seated neurosis based on the fact that your parents used food as a reward and punishment for your academic performance. What is it—anorexia, bulimia, binge-eating disorder?"

"No, I'm having guests over and I just wanted some dessert."

I finally felt as though I could be of some assistance.

"Ma'am, I know exactly what you need."

I reached into the display case and grabbed a hazelnut mocha cake and half a dozen fresh apple turnovers. I handed her the box of baked goods, sneered at Leyner, and added, "*This* is the perfect cure."

Why do they call it your funny bone if it hurts so bad?

Now, this is some serious medical humor. The "funny bone" refers to the superficial site where the ulnar nerve crosses the elbow. The name funny bone apparently came from a pun in the 1800s. It's a play on the word humorous and the upper arm bone, the humerus.

Try and contain your laughter.

The pain that you get from banging the funny bone occurs when you bang the nerve against the bony prominence of the humerus, the medial condyle. A simple bang of the elbow is painful, but there are some severe problems that can come from injuring this vulnerable nerve. Cubital tunnel syndrome is a condition that is also known as ulnar nerve entrapment neuropathy at the elbow. This is the second most common condition where a peripheral nerve gets compressed. The most common is carpal tunnel syndrome.

Ulnar nerve entrapment neuropathy at the elbow typically has an insidious onset—the cubital tunnel syndrome causes numbness in the ring and small fingers of the hand, elbow pain, and hand weakness. The symptoms are worsened by any activity that involves repeated flexing of the elbow. It is three times more common in men than women. Sometimes it even requires a surgical decompression to take pressure off the nerve. Not so funny.

How does aspirin find the pain?

Aspirin is really a magical little pill and probably one of the most important medications available. Aspirin has a very powerful preventive effect associated with strokes and heart disease. But most of us know it for curing pain, and it's common for people to wonder just how aspirin knows how to find that aching area.

The answer is that it doesn't! Aspirin is not the pain-seeking bloodhound it appears to be. Pain is a very complex process, and although we would love to avoid an explanation, here is a simplified version ...

Let's say you're bowling with your friend Barney and you drop the bowling ball on your toe. Although the pain is felt in the throbbing toe, it is really processed in the brain. After the ball crushes the toe, the cells and nerve endings are damaged and release chemicals. These chemicals send messages along the pain fibers to the brain where they are registered as pain. One group of chemicals involved is called prostaglandins, and aspirin works by stopping the cells from making prostaglandins. Prostaglandins are also responsible for inflammation and aspirin also blocks this effect.

So now you need some pain medication. When you take aspirin, it is absorbed in the stomach or intestine and it enters the bloodstream. From there it goes throughout the entire body, not just the injured area. It works its magic wherever prostaglandins are being made. The result—temporary relief of pain and inflammation.

Why do feet smell?

The fancy term for smelly feet is bromohydrosis. Hyperhidrosis refers to sweaty feet. In our family, we call it "swamp foot."

Foot odor is caused primarily from sweat, and the feet contain an estimated quarter of a million sweat glands. Just as in the armpits, foot sweat is odor-free when it comes out, but the bacteria on the surface of the feet act on the sweat and the stink begins. It becomes more of an issue down there, because our shoes and socks create a dark and moist environment that allows the bacteria to flourish.

The two solutions to the smelly foot problem are to keep your feet clean and to keep them dry. In the ER, we have a lot of experience with smelly feet. When caring for a particularly unkempt patient, an experienced ER doctor or nurse knows that the smell gets worse when the socks come off. There is a special name for this condition—we call it "toxic-sock syndrome."

Does arthritis flair up in bad weather?

Here we go again. We know what's going to happen when we say that there is no relationship between weather changes and arthritis. It will happen on some obscure radio program in Scottsdale, Arizona. The host will take calls, and some angry senior will call in, get all indignant, and berate us about the misinformation that we are irresponsibly spreading. He will tell us how he was hobbled by arthritis while living in Walla Walla, Washington, but now plays three sets of tennis a day. When we explain that the research literature has found no connection, he will become even more incensed.

There is no conspiracy here. Studies that have looked at the subjective perception of pain have found that changes in barometric pressure have caused increased pain, decreased pain, or no change at all. There is no consistent pattern. When researchers tried to look at objective measures of inflammation with weather changes, no study was able to find any connection.

So whether you live in New York City; an Amazonian rainforest; Tucson, Arizona; New Jersey; or the Gobi Desert, science cannot predict any changes with your arthritis with the climate. Check them all out and see which locale you prefer. (We would choose New York—the take-out is better.)

Why does it feel so hot outside when it is 90 degrees if our body temperature is 98.6?

This is a great question that we have been asked many times. There is a relatively simple explanation.

It's all about the thermoregulation. Doesn't sound very simple, does it? That's why we're here. Our bodies are constantly producing heat from our metabolism. This heat needs to go somewhere. Thermoregulation is the mechanism by which our body attempts to balance heat gain and loss in order to maintain a constant body temperature. This becomes more complicated when we are dealing with rising outside temperatures. It is much easier to release this heat when there is a large gradient (a bigger difference) between body and outside temperature. When it is hot outside, the body ends up having to work harder to lose heat. That makes you sweat and flush, as you try to increase blood flow to the skin and allow heat loss.

This just goes with the territory of being the warm-blooded animals that we are. Cold-blooded animals only get as hot or as cold as it is outside— which could be trouble for a rattlesnake trapped in an ice-cream truck.

Why does sucking on helium make your voice sound funny?

Helium is a colorless, odorless noble gas. The noble moniker doesn't make sense when you imagine a grown man at a child's party taking a balloon, inhaling, and then giggling like a five-year-old when he hears his own squeaky cartoon-like voice.

Helium causes this voice change by altering the environment where sound is formed. In normal conditions, the voice makes sounds using the vocal cords. The cords or folds vibrate, releasing pulses or waves of air into the throat. These waves are interpreted as sound. If we change the composition of the air, we change the way the vocal cords vibrate. Helium is lighter than air so our vocal cords will vibrate faster in this environment. The speed of sound in air is approximately 350 m/s, but the speed of sound in helium is 900 m/s. The faster vibration causes the higher pitch.

List of our favorite high-pitched voices:

Tweety Bird
Tiny Tim
Alvin and the Chipmunks
Mike Tyson

What turns snot green?

People are obsessed with the color of their secretions. In the hospital, you often get detailed descriptions about the color changes in a person's stool, urine, or sputum. Stool color changes can reflect illness, but urine color is rarely helpful unless blood is present. As for snot, identifying the rainbow of possibilities may be helpful in some patients. Green is the only potentially worrisome shade. The green color comes from white blood cells called neutrophils. These immune cells appear when bacteria starts infecting the nasal passages or airways. When the white cells start fighting the infection, they produce an enzyme called myeloperoxidase. Myeloperoxidase is green because it contains a lot of iron.

Now, the hint of a green tinge doesn't necessarily mean that you need antibiotics. If it is just in your nose at the beginning of an illness, it will probably pass. But if you are coughing it up, have underlying lung disease, or symptoms persist, go see your doctor.

So don't take umbrage with people who blow their noses and then carefully inspect the tissue or handkerchief to evaluate their production. They are just being vigilant.

Why do older people fart more than younger people?

We tried to find the derivation of the expression "old fart" but were unsuccessful. We will have to assume that it has something to do with an older person's propensity to let his flatulence fly without any regard for where he is when he is passing wind.

There are some reasons why the elderly would be more flatulent than their younger counterparts. Even if older folks are not actually producing more intestinal gas, loss of muscle tone occurs with the aging process and this includes the muscles around the anal sphincter. Therefore, an older person has less ability to hold gas in.

Other suitably ripe euphemisms for flatulence include:

- cutting the cheese.
- sneezing in one's pants.
- floating an air biscuit.
- sphincter whistling.
- killing the canary.
- colon bowlin'.
- the scented scream.

Can bald men get lice?

So you are going bald, but trying to look on the bright side, right? You make a list of all the positives; no wasting time in the morning with hairstyling, less money spent on products, no more hat head, no dandruff, and of course, no head lice.

Well, you may not be so lucky. You don't have to worry about the styling, the hat head, or the typical head lice, but you might still have dandruff and there are other crawling creatures that could attack your bald scalp.

There are several different types of lice: head lice (*Pediculus humanus capitis*), body lice (*Pediculus humanus corporis*), and pubic lice (*Pthirus pubis*). Head lice are the most common of all lice and are often seen in the heads of schoolchildren. Pubic lice are often referred to as "crabs." Crabs are frequently spread by sexual contact, and body lice are most often found in people who don't wash or change clothes often. In the ER, we often see homeless patients who are unfortunately infested with body lice.

Head lice probably won't have anything to grab on to on the bald head, but body lice might spread to affect a bald head. Scabies is another creepy crawler that is often confused with body lice. Scabies is an infestation of the skin with the microscopic mite *Sarcoptes scabei*. These mites are much tinier than lice. You can get scabies from direct contact with a person already infested with scabies. Infestation can also occur from sharing clothing, towels, or bedding.

Do humans really use only 10 to 20 percent of their brains?

There are many different nonscientific answers to this question. A wife might argue that her husband uses less than 10 percent of his brain at times, a coach often tells his players that they aren't using their heads enough, and we often think that our politicians don't use their brains at all. The truth is that there is no way to quantify how much of our brains we use at any given time. Humans definitely use more than 10 to 20 percent of their brains, so this myth is definitely false.

We are getting closer to understanding how we use our brains. Functional magnetic resonance imaging (fMRI) is a new technique that is being used to investigate which parts of the brain are active during different mental activities. Functional MRI measures changes in blood flow within the brain in response to various stimuli.

This isn't a direct measure of brain-cell activity, but it gives us a better idea how the brain works.

So maybe someday we can place George Bush in a functional MRI and really find out what's going on inside his noggin.

Why do Asians turn red after consuming alcohol?

We thought about cutting this question because of the risk of sounding racist, but before anyone jumps to conclusions, go do some reading about the metabolism of alcohol and specifically the low-Km mitochondrial aldehyde dehydrogenase (ALDH2) isoenzyme.

Yes, that's right. There is a physiological reason why some Asians, including Chinese, Japanese, and Koreans, get flushed in the face after drinking alcohol.

Here's what happens: alcohol (ethanol) is metabolized in the liver. In the first step, it is broken down by an enzyme, alcohol dehydrogenase, and forms a toxic compound known as acetaldehyde. After that, a second enzyme called aldehyde dehydrogenase 2 (ALDH2) converts the acetaldehyde into acetic acid (the main component of vinegar), which is nontoxic and can be readily converted by your body to provide energy.

Certain Asians lack this second enzyme and the acetaldehyde builds up. The side effects include skin flushing, increased heart rate, and severe nausea and vomiting. The severity of these symptoms depends on the degree of the enzyme deficiency.

If you dream in color, does it mean you are crazy?

I dream in color. Mark, on the other hand, dreams in high-definition IMAX, and the dialogue in his dreams is dubbed in poorly synchronized staccato Portuguese. But this doesn't mean that either of us is crazy.

Dreaming in color is a perfectly normal phenomenon. Scientists have always reported that people dream in both color and black and white, but the concept that dreams were primarily in black and white evolved in the 1950s. At that time, television, movies, etc., were almost entirely in black and white, and this probably led to the false perception that dreaming also followed this monochromatic pattern.

In 1962, in an article in *Science*, Kahn, Dement, Fisher, and Barmack reported on the "Incidence of Color in Immediately Recalled Dreams." These researchers woke their subjects up from REM sleep, and asked them if they dreamed in color. Eighty-three percent of their dreamers reported dreaming in color, and then, presumably, went back to sleep.

Is it true that you cannot die in a dream?

So here is the myth: if you are having a dream and you are about to die or be killed, you better wake up.

If not, you will die in the dream and remain in that eternal slumber. The reality is that you can die in a dream and be perfectly okay. Death dreams are not extremely common, but they do occur.

There are, however, some reports of true "killer dreams." It is known that emotional stress can cause an increase in heart rate and that this can occur during sleep, especially in REM sleep when dreams occur. It is also known that approximately 20 percent of heart attacks and 15 percent of sudden cardiac deaths occur between midnight and 6 a.m. Now, not all of these events are sleep- or dream-related, but there may be some risk for those with underlying heart disease.

For those of us who are healthy of heart, an article in the *Canadian Journal of Cardiology* described four cases of people without known heart disease for whom the emotional stress of nightmares caused their premature demise.

So should we sleep with one eye open for fear of a death dream? No, we didn't intend to scare you; you are much more likely to have a wet dream than a death dream, so enjoy your sleep.

Are there more violent crimes when the moon is full?

We already dispelled a similar myth about more babies being conceived when the moon is full. This one has no basis in science either.

Several studies have examined lunar cycles and violent behavior. There is no scientific or statistical support for a connection between a full moon and aggressive or violent behavior.

Now, when Billy goes to the ER for his next overnight, and it just happens that the moon is full, there is no way he is going to convince anyone that there isn't a relationship. Sometimes we just need something to blame.

Are you more likely to die in the passenger seat in a car accident?

In the emergency room where Dr. Billy works, it is extremely common to see patients after a motor-vehicle crash. We use the term "crash" rather than "accident" because accidents should be avoidable. Seat-belt use clearly reduces the number of serious injuries, but is there a safer place to sit in the car?

The passenger seat is often the preferred travel seat, with a battle raging for who gets to ride "shot-gun." This term is a reference to the days when stage-coaches would frequently get held up and an armed guard would ride alongside the driver for protection. Others refer to the passenger seat as the "death seat" and this appellation has some truth behind it.

Several studies have confirmed that sitting in the

front seat of a car is more dangerous than riding in the back. Sitting in the back can reduce the risk of death in a motor-vehicle crash by anywhere from 25 to 39 percent. The risk of serious injury is also reduced by about 30 percent for those sitting in the rear when compared with the front-seat riders. The risk to drivers is about the same as for those who are riding shotgun.

The bottom line is that the "death seat" name is justified, it just applies to both positions up front. So take your choice, sit in back where it is safer or ride up front where you can play with the radio.

Either way, make sure to buckle up.

Is there such a thing as a death erection?

Some people think that when you die you're bathed in a radiant light, you go to heaven or to hell, or you take up residence in the bodies of other creatures like lemurs or llamas. Others think that when you die, the following occurs:

- Your blood will pool due to gravity (hypostasis).
- You will gradually stiffen due to a buildup of lactic acid in your muscles (rigor mortis).
- You will become bloated by the production of gases caused by bacterial breakdown of tissue.

Oh, we forgot to mention that for men who die

face down, the pooling of blood will lead to a death erection.

Yes, this myth is true!

Some refer to this phenomenon as "angel lust."

Rest in peace.

Why do you shiver after you pee?

There are probably many sophisticated and urbane women out there who don't know that it's fairly common for men to experience a little shiver just as they finish urinating. And there are probably just as many men out there who shiver after they pee, but don't have the foggiest notion as to why.

Now we're not talking about a cold-induced shiver here … the camping-in-the-Arctic-and-taking-an-early-morning-whizz-in-the-woods shiver. We're talking about something a wee bit more mysterious …

Although this is a common male physiological phenomenon, there has been, to our knowledge, no scientific research conducted to explain its basis.

It is thought, though, that the pee shiver is related to the autonomic nervous system (ANS). The sympathetic subdivision of the ANS keeps the bladder relaxed and the urethral sphincter contracted so we don't wet our pants during an episode of fight-or-flight anxiety. When you go, the parasympathetic side of the ANS causes a contraction of the bladder and a relaxation of the urethral sphincter, enabling you to take a piss.

Dr. R. James Swanson, professor of biological sciences at Old Dominion University—and one of the only scientists intrepid and curious enough to publicly weigh in on the subject—muses that "The sympathetic outflow of action potential … would include the release of the adrenal medulla catacholamines epinephrine, norepinephrine and dopamine. When the opportunity arises to allow the parasympathetic side of the ANS to take over, the change in catacholamine production might be the cause of the shiver." Dr. Swanson adds that, in addition to the shiver, you will also notice a momentary "euphoria" shortly after relaxing the urethral sphincter.

Some yoga-oriented folks have compared the pee shiver to an orgasmic Kundalini energy flow. And the term "mini-orgasm" comes up with surprising frequency in discussions of this simultaneously mundane and esoteric subject.

Leyner and I think the fact that a man could have a quasiorgasmic response to merely relaxing his urethral sphincter shows just how ridiculously easy we are.

1:25 p.m.
Gberg: Leyner!!!
Leyner: WHAT?????!!!!!!!!!

Gberg: Don't throw all those question marks at me.

Leyner: Sorry.

Leyner: This day is whack.

Gberg: Why?

Leyner: So much bullshit to deal with on Mondays.

Gberg: Tell me why you don't like Mondays.

Gberg: Just checked Amazon and Barnes and Noble again ...

Leyner: Mondays ... just lots of stuff to attend to, and e-mails that piled up, and house stuff ...

Gberg: 217 and 235.

Leyner: That's nice.

1:30 p.m.

Leyner: I'm gonna call Carrie this week and talk to her about the schedule and deadline.

Gberg: I also was scouring the reviews. I can't control myself.

Gberg: We can talk to her tomorrow.

Leyner: I know you can't.

Leyner: I want to tell her that we might need a couple of extra weeks.

Gberg: I still want a piece of that guy who called the book mindless pablum.

Leyner: Let's find out where he lives.

Gberg: He wrote "It's a dough-grab attempt to top the *NY Times* best-seller list by appealing to jackasses."

Gberg: How dare he insult the jackasses that buy this book!

Leyner: I like that phrase: "dough-grab."

Leyner: I guess I should go work some more ... I want to do some more research ... I'm trying to gather all the stuff on puberty ... and then write them up. I wanna get the funny kicker to your peeing question done and the goose bump q and a for the catalog too. I'm also trying to get some work done each day on my script.

1:35 p.m.

Gberg: Script?

Leyner: Script.

Gberg: I thought you were dedicated 100% to *Why Do Men Fall Asleep After Sex?*

Leyner: The script I have to write ... that's due by the end of April.

Leyner: I am. Just trying to lay some groundwork so I can get that finished in time.

Gberg: I know what it is. I feel like you are cheating on me.

Gberg: Brutus.

Leyner: I'm not writing it. Just trying to begin to get some idea of what the movie is ... Don't ever call me a Brutus again.

Leyner: I'm really the most loyal person you'll ever know.

Gberg: I meant Brutus from the *Popeye* cartoons, not Caesar's Brutus.

Gberg: I would never question your loyalty. You are freakin' sensitive today.

Leyner: I'm feeling a little slammed today ... I'm completely sleep-deprived today ... I really got NONE. I looked at the clock and it was 4 am and I hadn't slept at all yet and I figured it was a little late for sleeping pills ... so I just read my Lord Nelson book until it was time to get my daughter ready for school.

Gberg: Take care of yourself. Take a nap.

Leyner: I'm twitchy and misanthropic and needing to be held and loved and fellated by burger waitresses.

Gberg: Burger waitresses? Are you thinking about that girl who served us last week? I didn't know she made such an impression.

Leyner: I thought she was mighty fine.

1:45 p.m.

Leyner: There was a big *Nipples* extract today in the *Daily Express* in England.

Gberg: I refuse to get into a discussion of what you want to do to yourself with burger waitresses. Then we will get more bad reviews on Amazon. Like the guy who called us arrogant and witless.

Gberg: I heard that there was also a two-page story in *Yediot Achronot* (Israel's #1 daily newspaper).

Leyner: Arrogant AND witless. Gosh ... he makes

us sound like brown-shirted fascists.

Leyner: Really, in *Yediot Achronot*?

Leyner: Does that mean idiotic spider in Hebrew?

Gberg: We also got "Mindless alcoholic ramblings," "Not worth the buy."

Gberg: I am so obsessed with the bad reviews I have them all saved in one Word document.

Leyner: Mindless alcoholic ramblings??? You sure he wasn't reading my other books?

Gberg: I wish I could e-mail him and suggest it.

Leyner: That's funny. You should.

Gberg: It was probably my ex who wrote that.

Leyner: Hey ... guess I should go and do something productive ... collate my notes about pilo-erection.

1:50 p.m.

Leyner: I'll call you after the interviews are over, OK?

Gberg: You know piloerection is a sign of heroin/opiate withdrawal.

Leyner: It's also a symptom of temporal lobe epilepsy and autonomic hyperreflexia.

Gberg: You go, girl!

Leyner: Thanks, sweetheart. Later, baby.

Gberg: Ciao.

Why does my butt itch so much?

If you are a sufferer of pruritus ani (itchy anus), you will relate to this question. Nobody likes to talk about it, but many of us know about the overwhelming, irresistible urge to scratch. It often happens at night and after a scratch and sniff, you are faced with one of the age-old dilemmas. Do you get out of bed and wash your smelly fingers?

Pruritus ani is a real and common condition. It is a chronic itching of the skin around the anus. The skin in that area becomes irritated from digestive products in the stool and this leads to an itchy rash. Excessive wiping or scrubbing with soap and water can make it even worse.

For simple solutions, avoid further trauma to the area (no scratching, no scrubbing), don't use soap of any kind on the anal area, and when wiping, use wet toilet paper, baby wipes, or a wet washcloth to blot the area clean.

Other things can cause itching in the perianal area including psoriasis, hemorrhoids, fungal infections, and pinworm. So if your itching persists, don't be embarrassed at being bare-assed. Go see your doctor.

What causes a split stream when you pee?

The International Classification of Diseases, Ninth Revision, Clinical Modification (ICD-9-CM) is the official system of assigning codes to diagnoses associated with hospitals in the United States. In case you wanted to know, the code for splitting of the urinary stream is 788.61.

The split stream is a real condition, but this code doesn't apply to you if you just occasionally wake up and pee in all directions like a sprinkler before it coalesces into a smooth even flow. This is probably caused by some residual debris in the urinary tube (urethra). Persistent split stream can be caused by a scarring of the urinary opening (meatal stenosis) or damage to the urethra. Prostate infections or enlargement of the prostate can also cause splitting of your flow.

So, if this problem persists, go see the urologist—and, guys, remember to lift up the seat (and don't forget to put it back down)!

• Chapter 12 •

'Tis the Season (to Ask Questions)

I t was a classic holiday evening in New York. Snow was gently falling, Bing Crosby music was playing, and Wendy was cleaning and decorating the office for the small party that we had planned to celebrate the season. Our exclusive guest list included Leyner and his lovely wife, Mercedes; me and my wonderful wife, Jessica; and Wendy and her new boyfriend, Dexter, the guy from the bakery. Their relationship had unexpectedly blossomed after Leyner thrust them together.

The six of us were gathered in the office and I had raised my glass to toast our prosperous first year in practice, when I heard a knock at the door and then the harmonious sounds of Christmas carolers singing "Silent Night." Leyner went to open the door. There was a large group of merry, red-cheeked people who entered. I was so stunned that it took me a moment to focus and recognize that these new guests were all patients of ours. There was the couple with the marital problems, Judd Wilson with his body-image issues, Stanislav Javenuski, the crying hockey player, the chess-playing chimp and his companion, Isabel Collier and her husband with their newborn baby, little Richard and his singing family, the miniature-golfing Japanese gangsters, and Ralph and Cindy Tucker and their pubescent daughter, Stacey.

I pulled Leyner aside angrily. "Do you have an explanation for this? You are breaking every single rule of patient confidentiality."

"Lighten up, Scrooge. I got you something."

Leyner reached into his ever-present Yak Pak—the black bag he carries with him everywhere—and pulled out a wrapped gift.

"Happy Hanukah, *mon frère*."

I shook my head, constantly amazed at these unexpected instances of Leyner's generosity and good nature.

"And I have something for you too, *hermano*."

We exchanged gifts and immediately tore at the wrapping paper.

I'd gotten Leyner an expensive and rare first edition of Robert Louis Stevenson's *Dr. Jekyll and Mr. Hyde* in honor of the strange dynamic of our working relationship.

When I unwrapped Leyner's gift, I found myself holding a glazed ceramic decanter in the shape of a genie's bottle. The cap was an exact scale replica of Leyner's head. The bottle was filled with some foul-looking liquid. Overcome with curiosity, I unscrewed the

Leyner "head," and carefully wafted the bouquet toward my nose. The acrid aroma burned my nostrils.

"What the hell is that?!"

Leyner smiled, winking at me. "I reformulated and tweaked the recipe. It's MegaProfen-11™. You're going to love it, dude!"

Wendy poured paper cupfuls of MegaProfen-11™ for all the guests. With cups raised, I began my toast …

"Here's to a glorious year and special appreciation to all of you who sought out our guidance. It means so much that you had the confidence and trust to allow us into your lives. We have learned as much from you as we hope you have learned from us. *Salud*."

Are poinsettia plants really poisonous?

With all that yummy stuff to eat during the Christmas season, like roast goose and baked ham, it's a bit of a mystery to us why anyone would eat poinsettia plants. But people do seem to pass on the fruitcake and reach for the *Euphorbia pulcherrima* (that's poinsettia for those of you who are botanically challenged). In the 2004 annual report of the American Association of Poison Control Centers Toxic Exposure Surveillance System, 2,206 poinsettia exposures were reported to poison-control centers.

Here's the lowdown on the poinsettia chow-down. It's not going to kill you. Rumors of the lethal effects of the plant probably started back in 1919, when the two-year-old child of a U.S. army officer was thought to have died after ingesting poinsettia leaves. Upon investigation by the American Society of Florists, though, it was determined that the leaves were not responsible for the death of this child. But the misconception about the poisonous nature of this much-maligned plant has persisted. A recent study by Children's Hospital of Pittsburgh and Carnegie Mellon University determined that out of some 23,000 reported poinsettia exposures, there was essentially no toxicity of any kind.

If you're heedlessly herbivorous, plan on eating the mistletoe after kissing your sweetheart underneath. That's not toxic either.

Can you get Lyme disease from a reindeer?

It looks like Santa's elves might need to start checking each other for ticks. Leyner and I were unable to find a case report of an elf afflicted with Lyme disease, but we offer the following scientific analysis and deductive reasoning—Lyme disease is caused by the bacterium *Borrelia burgdorferi* and is transmitted by the bite of infected ticks. In the northeast of the United States, *Ixodes dammini* (the deer tick) is the chief carrier of this disease. Thus, we implicate deer in the spread of the ailment.

Now for the reindeer connection. Reindeer (*Rangifer tarandus*)—otherwise known as caribou—are medium-sized members of the deer family. Reindeer are found in many regions of the world, including Sweden. Guess what else is commonly found in Sweden? Buxom blond women eating pickled herring? Yes, that's correct, but that has absolutely nothing to do with deer ticks. Guess again … Time's up! You are correct, sir! Lyme disease. We also know that moose and roe deer, among other large mammals in Sweden, are vectors for Lyme disease. So it makes perfect sense that Dasher, Blitzen, and Rudolph might also be complicit.

Why does turkey make you so sleepy?

You have just scarfed down several pounds of turkey, a terrine full of mashed potatoes, 8 ounces of tangy cranberry sauce, half a green-bean casserole, and several large hunks of fruitcake. And you wonder why you just fell asleep on the couch in front of the TV, as your uncle Howard drones on soporifically yet again about his chance encounter with some second-rate actor on a Florida golf course five decades ago.

It's very common for people to report drowsiness after eating the traditional Christmas meal. And it's equally common for the armchair expert in the family to blame it on the turkey and the tryptophan. L-tryptophan is an amino acid that helps the body produce the B vitamin niacin, which promotes the production of serotonin, a neurotransmitter that acts as a calming agent in your brain.

L-tryptophan is naturally found in turkey protein, but a typical serving of turkey contains a similar amount of L-tryptophan as found in an average serving of chicken and minced meat. So it's probably not the turkey.

It's most likely that the enormity of the meal itself is precipitating that postprandial prostration. Christmas gluttony causes a variety of digestive substances to jump into action and ultimately leads to increased blood flow and metabolic rate for digestion.

What was wrong with Tiny Tim in *A Christmas Carol*?

Tiny Tim Cratchit is one of the most poignant characters in the history of Christmas literature and movies. For many people, he is the very embodiment of physical disability, and few can forget his sweet and saintly disposition. He represented for author Charles Dickens the wretched state of children in Victorian England. What actually afflicted this character, though, and made him dependent on that crutch and hideous frame of metal and leather on his legs and lower back?

Although Dickens never reveals specifically what ails the poor, undersized lad, medical experts generally have three opinions. Tiny Tim possibly suffered from distal renal tubular acidosis (type 1), a disorder that is characterized by growth failure, and, left untreated, will result in fractures, muscle weakness, and ultimately kidney failure and death. This is an uncommon disease. The two other possibilities were much more prevalent at the time that Dickens wrote his classic tale. Rickets, a vitamin-D deficiency, would have resulted in Tiny Tim's soft bones, muscle weakness, and stunted growth. It has also been speculated that Tiny Tim was afflicted by Pott's disease, which is tuberculosis of the spine.

Thanks to the reformed Scrooge's redemptive revelations, Tiny Tim is granted a new lease of life and given the opportunity to celebrate Christmases Yet to Come. "God bless us, every one!"

Is it true that there are more suicides during the Christmas season?

We hate to say this as writers, but you shouldn't always believe what you read. The press and electronic media have persistently promulgated the myth that Americans are more likely to kill themselves at Thanksgiving, Christmas, and New Year's than at any other time of the year. Over 30 percent of news reports on the subject still disseminate this misinformation. The myth is fueled by a kind of counter-intuitive logic that severely depressed people become even more deeply depressed during this period of enforced good cheer. Not only does this turn out false, but there are actually fewer suicides during the holiday season than other times of the year. Data collected by the National Center for Health Statistics indicates that suicide rates are actually at their lowest in December, while peaking in the spring and fall. The speculation is that, at holiday time, people with a tendency toward depression have a stronger support system of family and friends than they would otherwise.

Can your tongue get stuck on a frozen pole?

Do you remember the classic 1983 movie *A Christmas Story*, in which nine-year-old Ralph "Ralphie" Parker and his loyal friend Flick are faced with a "triple-dog-dare," and poor Flick ends up sticking his tongue to a frozen flagpole until the fire department comes to the rescue?

What's the scientific explanation for this classic frozen faux pas? It's simple. Metal is a very good conductor of cold, and on a frigid winter's day, it's likely that most metal objects outside—including fences and mailboxes—are cold enough to reach temperatures that are significantly below freezing. If you're enough of a blockhead to actually accept this triple-dog-dare, here's what will happen. When you put your moist tongue against the frozen metal surface, the moisture on your tongue rapidly freezes and sticks to the metal.

If the quaint stupidity of this practice really appeals to you, buy the action figure. Yes, that's right! There's a Flick figure that comes with a "frozen" flagpole that magnetically attracts Flick's outstretched tongue. That way you can get all of the pleasure, with none of the pain.

Can you get drunk from eating Christmas cake?

A couple of shots of Jack Daniels and a beer will do the trick much more efficiently. But if you want to drown your sorrows in Christmas cake made with alcohol (or a sherry trifle), it all depends on how you prepare it and how much you eat. Here's a chart of the percentage of alcohol left in dishes following various methods of preparation.

Preparation Method	Alcohol Retained
Alcohol added to boiling liquid, and removed from heat	85%
Alcohol flamed	75%
No heat, stored overnight	70%
Baked, 25 minutes, alcohol not stirred into mixture	45%
Baked or simmered, alcohol stirred into mixture:	
15 minutes	40%
30 minutes	35%
1 hour	25%
1.5 hours	20%
2 hours	10%
2.5 hours	5%

Source: U.S. Department of Agriculture

After perusing several reliable Christmas-cake recipes, we found that you usually put in about a half cup of alcohol and bake for approximately one hour. In the end, there'd probably be less than an ounce of alcohol left in the entire cake. So you'd have to have either a very low tolerance for alcohol or the capacity to consume an outlandish amount of baked goods to get hammered on Christmas cake.

What would happen if a morbidly obese man got stuck in a chimney?

This question is an obvious attempt to diss Santa Claus.

First of all, Santa's ability to nimbly traverse rooftops, and maneuver himself down and then back up chimney stacks and through flues, hearths, and fireplaces of all sorts—all the while carrying an enormously heavy bag of gifts—obviously demonstrates an athleticism and an agility for a big man that belies the very meaning of "morbidly obese." (The term "morbidly obese" is applicable to people who are 50 to 100 percent—or 100 pounds—above their ideal body weight OR who have a body mass index value greater than thirty-nine.)

At a juncture in his career, when you'd expect him to be slowing down, Santa is actually putting up mind-boggling stats that surpass anything he's achieved thus far. Just compare him with other mythic icons, like Hercules or Popeye, at similar stages in their lives. After completing his record-breaking 12th

Labor (bringing Cerberus up from Hades), Hercules, by his own admission, was unable to maintain the intense drive that had distinguished his career. Popeye, of course, retired and opened up the American fast-food restaurant chain Popeye's.

During Christmas 2005, Santa delivered some 3.9 billion toys, shattering the mark he'd set the previous season. This has, predictably, fueled scurrilous and completely unsubstantiated rumors of steroid use.

For the record, Santa Claus has adamantly denied ever using steroids or performance-enhancing drugs of any kind, and he has offered to submit himself to year-round random testing.